I0767135

# Pioneer F.H.I.T

# Pioneer F.H.I.T

*Functional High Intensity Training*

Hashim Evans, Lmt, Sis, Lfc.

Copyright © 2019 by Hashim Evans, Lmt, Sis, Lfc.

ISBN:          Softcover                978-1-7960-1621-5
               eBook                    978-1-7960-1620-8

All rights reserved. No part of this book may be reproduced or transmitted in any form or by any means, electronic or mechanical, including photocopying, recording, or by any information storage and retrieval system, without permission in writing from the copyright owner.

The views expressed in this work are solely those of the author and do not necessarily reflect the views of the publisher, and the publisher hereby disclaims any responsibility for them.

Any people depicted in stock imagery provided by Getty Images are models, and such images are being used for illustrative purposes only.
Certain stock imagery © Getty Images.

Print information available on the last page.

Rev. date: 03/26/2019

**To order additional copies of this book, contact:**
Xlibris
1-888-795-4274
www.Xlibris.com
Orders@Xlibris.com
791927

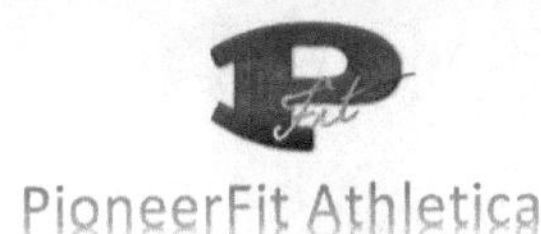


## Monday Workout

1- *6 minute warm up*
2- *Repeat the FHIT circuit 2 times each movement is for 1min*
3- *Take 2min to recover after completing FHIT circuit*
4- *After final break and completing both rounds do the 10min cool down.*

## Tuesday workout

1- *30min activity such as yoga or stretching*
2- *some use this as another cardio day*

## Wednesday Workout

1- *6 minute warm up*
2- *Repeat the FHIT circuit 2 times each movement is for 1min*
3- *Take 2min to recover after completing FHIT circuit*
4- *After final break and completing both rounds do the 10min cool down*

## Cardio
## Thursday workout

1- *6min warm up*
2- *30min of cardiovascular activity of your choice*
3- *10min of stretching*

## Pioneer Fit Power Circuit
## Friday workout

1- *warm up 6 min*
2- *6min is all that's needed for this workout, continuous clock*
3- *12 reps each exercise one after the next until the time is up*

## <u>Workout break down as follows:</u>

- *FHIT Circuit 2 day per week Monday, Wednesday*
- *Pioneer Power circuit 1 day per week Friday*
- *Full cardio day 1 day per week Thursday*
- *Full recovery flexibility/ Stretching Tuesday*

Bonus 4-week pre-training

This 4-week pre-training program will improve your strength and cardio fitness, it will prepare your body to safely tackle the main workout program. Each workout in pre-training will condition all parts of the body, including legs, core and arms. the pre-training program includes FHIT circuit training, a weekly pioneer power up workout, recovery session and cardio. There are less jumping exercises compared to the main program, so you can concentrate on overall conditioning.

## 12-WEEK STEP BY STEP FITNESS GUIDE-BURN FAT AND RE-INVENT YOUR SHAPE

- RAPIDLY BURN FAT WITH OUR HIGH INTENSITY PROGRAM
- WORKOUT ANYTIME, ANYWHERE, WITH NO EQUIPMENT
- VERY STRUCTURED PROGRAM
- YOU WILL FEEL THE AMAZING DIFFERENCE IN 2 WEEKS
- VERY SIMPLE TO FOLLOW

## 5 REASONS YOU NEED TO TRY OUR FHIT BODY PROGRAM

1. OUR F.H.I.T BODY SYSTEM DELIVERS HUGE RESULTS IN A VERY SHORT AMOUNT OF TIME. IT WILL ACCELERATE FAT LOSS, BURN CALORIES ASWELL AS IMPROVE YOUR OVERALL FITNESS.
2. THE MAXIMUM AMOUNT OF TIME NEEDED IS 20 MINUTES, 3 TIMES A WEEK TO SEE RESULTS WITH A PROPER DIET. DURING THE PROGRAM, THE EXERCISES INCREASE IN INTENSITY AND

BECOME MORE COMPLEX AS YOUR FITNESS LEVEL INCREASES. AT THE END OF THIS PROGRAM YOU WILL SEE A MORE LEAN AND TONED IMAGE.

3. GET READY TO BE INTRODUCED TO YOUR F.H.I.T BODY. THE F.H.I.T BODY PROGRAM USES COMPOUND MOVEMENTS TO INCORPERATE AS MANY MUSCLE GROUPS AS POSSIBLE TO ACCELERATE FAT LOSS.

4. OUR STEP BY STEP GUIDE IS VERY EASY TO FOLLOW. THERE'S NO FITNESS EQUIPMENT NEEDED, AND NO EXPENSIVE GYM MEMBERSHIPS.

5. THE F.H.I.T BODY PROGRAM IS DESIGNED FOR BUSY PEOPLE LIKE YOU, TO ACHIEVE OPTIMUM RESULTS IN THE SHORTEST AMOUNT OF TIME. THE EXERCISES CAN BE DONE ANYWHERE, THE BEDROOM, BEACH, OR EVEN THE BACK YARD. IN OTHER WORDS, ANYWHERE YOU CAN SPARE 20 MINUTES.

WHATS IN THE FHIT BODY PROGRAM?

12 WEEK FITNESS PROGRAM
- THE 12 WEEK FHIT PROGRAM IS FULL OF FUN, CHALLENGING, HIGH INTENSITY MOVEMENTS SURE TO KEEP YOU BURNING CALORIES.

OPTIMIZED TRAINING
- OUR TRAINING PROGRAM CONSISTS OF 4, 3 WEEK CYCLES. THIS IS DESIGNED TO HELP YOU REACH OPTIMAL PERFORMANCE, FITNESS, POWER AND FAT BURNING LEVELS.

SELECTIVE EXERCISE COMBINTATIONS FOR BEST RESULTS
- IN THE FHIT PROGRAM THE EXERCISES RANGE FROMBODY WEIGHT RESISTANCE EXERCISES, TO

JUMPING (PLYOMETICS) EXERCISES, CARDIO AND UNILATERAL MOVEMENTS.

## HIGH INTENSITY TRAINING CIRCUITS
- THE FUNCTIONAL HIGH INTENSITY TRAINING CIRCUITS ARE SAFE, MAXIMIZE POWER AND FAT BURNING.

## THE PIONEER WORKOUTS
- A 6 MINUTE EXPLOSIVE WORKOUT TO PUSH 100% EFFORT AND TRAIN THE BODY AT A DEEP LEVEL.

## FHIT TIPS
- TIPS TO HELP LOSE WEIGHT AND TO ACCELERATE FAT LOSS.

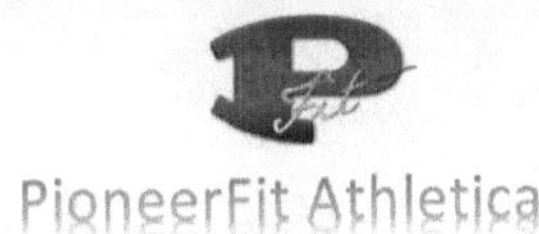

# Legal disclaimer:

Pioneer Fit Athletica LLC developed the Pioneer Fit shred method, however we are not a medical organization and cannot provide you any medical advice. We strongly urge you to consult with your physician before starting on any exercise or diet plan.

The Pioneer Fit shred program is designed to improve your health but is not intending to treat any illness or disease. If you choose to follow the Pioneer fit shred program without consulting your physician, you are doing so at your own risk.

We claim no responsibility for any injuries you might sustain. Exercises include detailed descriptions to give you the information you need to be able to perform the exercise with proper form. However, it is your responsibility to warm up properly. It is up to you to determine if you can perform the exercise/ workout without sustaining injury.

There are no guarantees as to outcomes. Our personal methods of training and weight loss, while solely created and tested by us, are not intended to convey any warranty, either expressed or implied, as to outcomes, promises or benefits.

The 3 biggest benefits of the FHIT program

- BURN FAT RAPIDLY - SCULPT YOUR BODY - SAVE TIME & MONEY

## <u>BURNING FAT RAPIDLY</u>

The FHIT method switches your body into hyperdrive to super charge your fat loss and jump start your metabolism. The goal is to push your body into the anaerobic zone with high intensity circuits. Working at maximum effort for short, explosive bursts your body falls into oxygen debt. This oxygen debt will be repaid post work out in the form of a boost to your metabolism resulting in a higher calorie burn.

## <u>SCULPT YOUR BODY</u>

Have you ever been on a diet? If so you have probably been frustrated with losing muscle along with fat. The FHIT program has the unique ability to burn fat fast while preserving lean muscle. In as little as 2 weeks, you will start to see improvements in your lean muscle and overall shape.

## <u>SAVE TIME & MONEY</u>

The FHIT program is perfect for busy people who want convenience as well as results. Our workouts can be done anytime, anywhere with minimal equipment. With our program there is no need for a gym membership or trainer.

### <u>Unique Exercise Combination</u>

With our interesting and unique blend of bodyweight resistance movements, plyometrics and unilateral exercises, combined into each training circuit. Stimulating as many muscles groups as possible, to accelerate fat loss and improve overall fitness. Throw in a cardio session weekly, some recovery time and you will be in the best shape of your life.

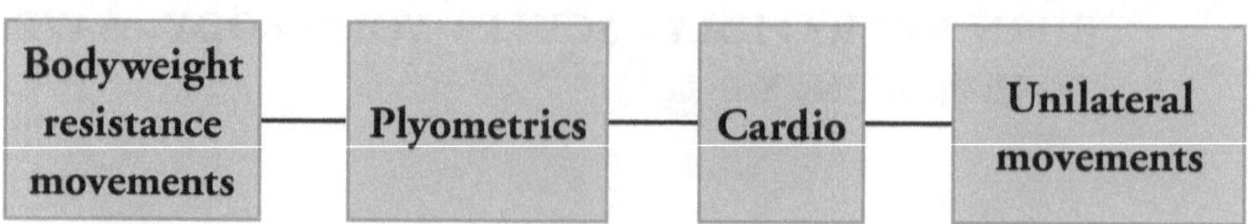

## Plyometric movements

- Plyometrics are also known as jump training and or plyo's for short. These movements are explosive movements designed to build strength, speed and coordination. In plyometric exercises, your muscles are required to rapidly stretch and contract when jumping and landing. Popular with athletes, these exercises are designed to maximize performance, help you jump and run.

## Bodyweight Resistance

- Bodyweight Resistance movements are very simple yet effective. There is no equipment or weights required. In this program you use your very own bodyweight as the sole form of resistance. It is truly amazing what you can accomplish using just your bodyweight. Some examples of bodyweight movements are pushups, sit ups, squats, lunges etc. Bodyweight Movements helps produce core strength, balance as well as muscular endurance. Each movement selected in this program recruits multiple muscle groups for example, a squat is known to work your glutes, but it hits the quads, adductors, calves, hip flexors and core as well.

## Cardio

- aerobic or cardio exercises relies on the heart to shuttle oxygen to your muscles and raises your heart rate for an extended period. Cardio movements are included in any of our FHIT circuits to help the body recover and keep the heart pumping between the more intense exercises such as, jump rope and or lateral shuffles. In our program the designated day for cardio is Thursday, where you can choose to go for a brisk walk, jogging, swimming, spinning etc.

## Unilateral movements

- Unilateral exercises work one side of the body at a time and are ideal for improving balance and evening out any strength imbalances. You may not know if you favor your left or right side, but this kind of training will quickly reveal the truth. Unilateral movements like lunges and plank rotations require more balance and skill than the traditional bilateral exercises like squats.

## Program breakdown
### The FHIT Circuit

- Every Monday and Wednesday, you will complete a functional, High Intensity circuit that pushes the body to a different level. These workouts will hit the entire body but focus on upper body one day and lower body emphasis on the other. With exercises alternating between body parts as well as utilizing core strength maximum calories are expended.

## Cardio

- The cardio workout has a prescribed time limit, but less structure. You have the freedom to choose the type of cardio you want to complete, to fit in with your lifestyle and preferences. Cardio sessions are completed every Thursday and workouts can include brisk walk, jogging, swimming, cycling, using a cross trainer or indoor rower, or take a fitness class.

## The Pioneer-Power circuit

- Maximum effort is crucial to the success of any high intensity workout program. It is non-negotiable to achieve the best results.

## _THE JOURNEY_
## _BONUS PRE-TRAINING PROGRAM_

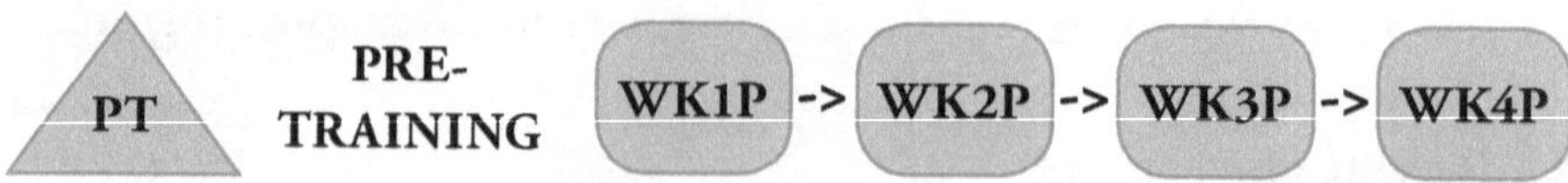

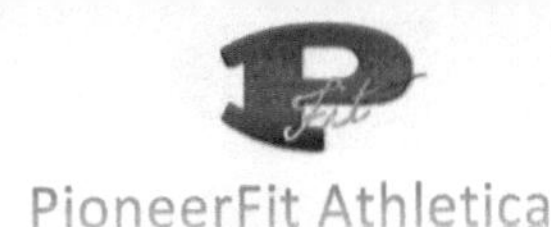


## *12- WEEK FITNESS PROGRAM*

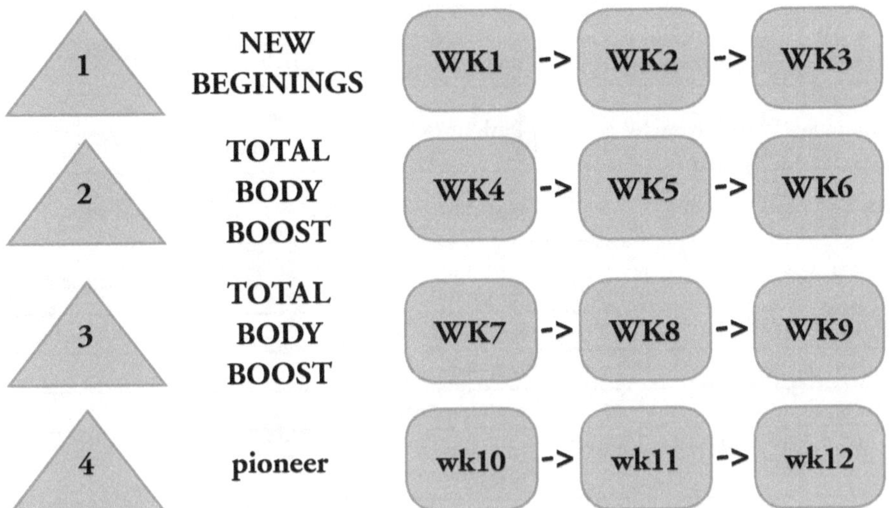


## *WARM UP EXERCISE CIRUIT: EACH MOVEMENT IS 30SEC EACH COMPLETE THE CIRCUIT 3X*

| 1ST ROUND SLOW | 2ND ROUND FASTER | 3RD ROUND FASTEST |
| --- | --- | --- |
| JOG IN PLACE | JOG IN PLACE | JOG IN PLACE |
| JUMPING JACKS | JUMPING JACKS | JUMPING JACKS |
| WIDE TIRE RUN | WIDE TIRE RUNS | WIDE TIRE RUNS |
| BUTT KICKS | BUTT KICKS | BUTT KICKS |

## *COOL DOWN STRETCHES THAT SHOULD BE DONE AFTER EACH WORKOUT:*

*Hamstring stretches- toe touches*
*Quadriceps/hip flexor stretches- pull heel to butt*
*Oblique stretches- lateral bends*
*Calf stretch-hang heel off step*
*Shoulder stretch- arms behind back*
*Abdominal stretch- cobra or sphinx*

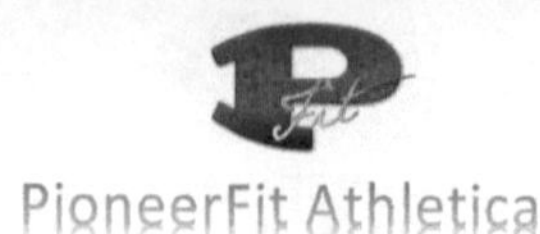



# Week 1 pre-training

| Monday F.H.I.T | Tuesday Recovery | Wednesday F.H.I.T | Thursday full cardio | Friday power |
|---|---|---|---|---|
| Sumo squats x30 | **Stretching** | Push-ups x20 | **Cardio 20-30minutes** | sumo squats x12 |
| High knees x1m | | glute bridges x30 | | pushup x12 |
| Leg scissors x25 | | walking lunges x40 | | ab bicycle x12 |
| Butt kicks x1m | | half burpee x20 | | high knees x12 |
| Triceps dips x25 | | oblique twist x40 | | |
| Ab bicycle x30 | | high knee x1m | | |
| Side shuffles x1m | | jumping jacks x50 | | |

# Week 2 pre-training

| Monday F.H.I.T | Tuesday Recovery | Wednesday F.H.I.T | Thursday full cardio | Friday power |
|---|---|---|---|---|
| walking lunge x30 | **Stretching** | Push-ups x30 | cardio 20m | alternating lateral lunge x12 |
| side shuffle 1m | | alternating lateral lunges | | half burpees x12 |
| leg lifts x25 | | half burpees x25 | | Russian twist x12 |
| plank jacks x40 | | ab bicycle x40 | | high knee x1m |
| superman x25 | | glute bridges x30 | | |
| heel raise x30 | | jumping jacks x50 | | |
| butt kicks x1m | | lateral shuffle x1m | | |

# Week 3 pre-training

| Monday F.H.I.T | Tuesday Recovery | Wednesday F.H.I.T | Thursday full cardio | Friday power |
|---|---|---|---|---|
| Sumo squats x30 | **Stretch** | Push-ups x20 | cardio 20min | sumo squat jumps x12 |

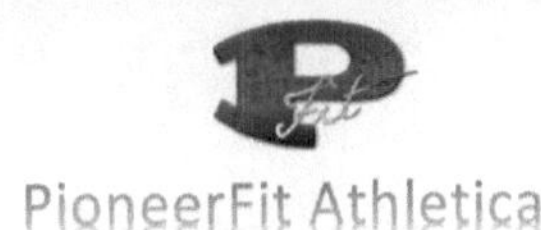



| High knees x1m | | glute bridges x30 | | pushup x12 |
|---|---|---|---|---|
| Leg scissors x25 | | walking lunges x40 | | ab bicycle x12 |
| Butt kicks x1m | | half burpee x20 | | high knees x12 |
| Triceps dips x25 | | oblique twist x40 | | |
| Ab bicycle x30 | | high knee x1m | | |
| Side shuffles x1m | | jumping jacks x50 | | |

## Week 4 pre-training

| Monday F.H.I.T | Tuesday Recovery | Wednesday F.H.I.T | Thursday full cardio | Friday power |
|---|---|---|---|---|
| walking lunge x30 | **Stretching** | Push-ups x30 | cardio 20m | alternating lateral lunge x12 |
| side shuffle 1m | | alternating side lunges | | half burpees x12 |
| leg lifts x25 | | half burpees x25 | | seated Russian twist x12 |
| plank jacks x40 | | ab bicycle x40 | | high knee x1m |
| superman x25 | | glute bridges x30 | | |
| heel raise x30 | | jumping jacks x50 | | |
| butt kicks x1m | | lateral shuffle x1m | | |

## Week 1, circuit 1

| Monday F.H.I.T | Tuesday Recovery | Wednesday F.H.I.T | Thursday full cardio | Friday power |
|---|---|---|---|---|
| Pioneer Squats | 10-minute Jump rope | 1. Mountain Climber | 30 min run | 1. Push up incline |
| Push ups | Basic stretches | 2. Stationary Lunges | | 2. 123 high knees |

| Squat Jumps | | 3. Burpee | | 3. In & out squat |
|---|---|---|---|---|
| Bench Dips | | 4. Glute Bridges | | 4. Bicycles |
| High Knee | | 5. bung | | |
| Bicycles | | 6. plank | | |
| Knee pulls | | 7. Hip rotations | | |

## Week 2, Circuit 2

| Monday F.H.I.T | Tuesday Recovery | Wednesday F.H.I.T | Thursday full cardio | Friday power |
|---|---|---|---|---|
| lateral shuffle | 10-minute jump rope | Bench dips | **Cardio** | lateral lunge |
| switch kicks | Basic stretches | In & Out Squats | | power jump |
| split jumps | | 123 Knee | | burpees |
| plank jacks | | lateral shuffles | | plank rotation |
| two pushups move | | Pushup jacks | | |
| squat touch turn | | Plank Alternating leg lift | | |
| Robot Pushups | | Bicycles | | |

## Week 3, Circuit 3

| Monday F.H.I.T | Tuesday Recovery | Wednesday F.H.I.T | Thursday full cardio | Friday power |
|---|---|---|---|---|
| Deep squats | 30min run | squat jumps | 10 min jump rope | glute bridges |
| Pushups | **Stretching** | high knees | | half burpee |
| Mountain climber | | push ups | | power jumps |
| Squat jumps | | plank lateral knee | | bungee |

| | | | | |
|---|---|---|---|---|
| High knees | | plank hip rotation | | |
| Half burpee | | 123 knees | | |
| Plank alter. arm lift | | walking lunges | | |

# Week 4, Circuit 4

| Monday F.H.I.T | Tuesday Recovery | Wednesday F.H.I.T | Thursday full cardio | Friday power |
|---|---|---|---|---|
| Split jump | **Stretching** | wide pushups | **30min cardio** | burpee |
| Lateral shuffle | | bungee | | pushup |
| 123 knees | | mountain climber | | plank hip rot |
| Pushup jack | | ladder climber | | plank jacks |
| Plank jacks | | power jumps | | |
| Plank alt. leg | | hi knee | | |
| Superman | | Bicycles | | |

# Week 5, Circuit 5

| Monday F.H.I.T | Tuesday Recovery | Wednesday F.H.I.T | Thursday full cardio | Friday power |
|---|---|---|---|---|
| sumo squat | 10 min jump rope | split jumps | 30min run | pushups |
| Walking lunge | **Stretching** | v ups | | plank jacks |
| Squat jumps | | plank alt leg lift | | bench dips |
| Split jumps | | back lunge | | superman |
| Glute bridge | | mountain climber | | |
| Power jumps | | Bungees | | |
| robot pushups | | plank alt knee | | |

# Week 6, Circuit 6

| Monday F.H.I.T | Tuesday Recovery | Wednesday F.H.I.T | Thursday full cardio | Friday power |
|---|---|---|---|---|
| Ski bump | **Stretching** | 2 pushups move | 30min run | power jump |

| front &<br>back hop | | Dips | | burpee |
|---|---|---|---|---|
| 123 knees | | plank alt leg | | towel jump |
| glute bridge | | plank arm lift | | plank alternating knee |
| back lunges | | half burpee | | |
| split jump | | mountain climb | | |
| robot pushup | | Bungees | | |

## Week 7, Circuit 7

| Monday<br>F.H.I.T | Tuesday<br>Recovery | Wednesday<br>F.H.I.T | Thursday full<br>cardio | Friday power |
|---|---|---|---|---|
| Forward and back hops | 30 min run | pushup inclined | jump rope | split jumps |
| Lateral lunges | **Stretching** | v ups | | v ups |
| Squat with side kick | | flutter kicks | | plank alt leg lift |
| Plank jacks | | mountain climb | | back lunge |
| Bungees | | Sumo Squats | | |
| Glute bridges | | bicycles | | |
| High knee | | sit through | | |

## Week 8, Circuit 8

| Monday<br>F.H.I.T | Tuesday<br>Recovery | Wednesday<br>F.H.I.T | Thursday full<br>cardio | Friday power |
|---|---|---|---|---|
| squat hold at bottom | jump rope | pushup hold | 30min run | split jump |
| split jump holds at bottom | **Stretching** | v ups hold | | front and back towel jump |
| high knee | | rotational mountain climber | | frog leap front/back |
| donkey 2sec hold | | superman holds | | high knees |
| Lateral towel jumps | | plank jacks | | |
| Back lunge hold | | bench dips | | |

| Squat front kick | | bicycle holds | | |
| --- | --- | --- | --- | --- |

## Week 9, Circuit 9

| Monday F.H.I.T | Tuesday Recovery | Wednesday F.H.I.T | Thursday full cardio | Friday power |
| --- | --- | --- | --- | --- |
| Ski bump holds | 30 min run | dips | jump rope | ski bump |
| In and out squats hold on out | **Stretching** | incline pushup | | squat front kick |
| plank jack | | plank shoulder taps | | Burpee |
| Alt back lunge | | plank hip rotation | | mountain climber |
| Squat jump | | dive bombers | | |
| Squat side kick | | v-ups | | |
| Leg scissors | | Bungee | | |

## Week 10, Circuit 10

| Monday F.H.I.T | Tuesday Recovery | Wednesday F.H.I.T | Thursday full cardio | Friday power |
| --- | --- | --- | --- | --- |
| Frog hops front & back | 10min jump rope | power jumps | 30min run | dips |
| Lateral lunge | **Stretching** | alt. front lunge | | wide pushup |
| Squat front kick | | half burpee | | dive bombers |
| Plank jacks | | in out squat | | Bicycles |
| Half burpee | | Bungees | | |
| Glute bridge | | alternating limb lifts | | |
| High knee | | plank rotation | | |

## Week 11, Circuit 11

| Monday F.H.I.T | Tuesday Recovery | Wednesday F.H.I.T | Thursday full cardio | Friday power |
| --- | --- | --- | --- | --- |
| lateral shuffle | 30 min run | Bench dips | **30 min cardio** | lateral lunge |
| switch kicks | **Stretching** | switch kicks | | power jump |
| split jumps | | 123 Knee | | Burpees |

| | | | | |
|---|---|---|---|---|
| plank jacks | | lateral shuffles | | plank rotation |
| two pushups move | | Pushup jacks | | |
| squat touch turn | | Plank Alternating leg lift | | |
| Robot Pushups | | bicycles | | |

# Week 12, Circuit 12

| Monday F.H.I.T | Tuesday Recovery | Wednesday F.H.I.T | Thursday full cardio | Friday power |
|---|---|---|---|---|
| Forward and back hops | 30 min run | pushup incline | jump rope | split jumps |
| Lateral lunges | **Stretching** | v ups | | v ups |
| Squat with side kick | | flutter kicks | | plank alt leg lift |
| Plank jacks | | mountain climb | | back lunge |
| Bungees | | squats | | |
| Glute bridges | | bicycles | | |
| High knee | | sit thru | | |

| Monday FHIT | TUESDAY CARDIO | WEDNESDAY FHIT | THURSDAY CARDIO | FRIDAY PIONEER POWER | |
|---|---|---|---|---|---|
| FHIT 2 X 7 MINUTE WORKOUT | | | | | |
| ✓ | | ✓ | | | |
| RECOVERY SESSION JUST MOVE STRETCHING & WALKING 30 MINUTES | | | | | |
| | ✓ | | | | |
| CARDIO SESSION 20 MINUTE OF EXERCISE | | | | | |
| | | | ✓ | | |
| PIONEER POWER UP WORKOUTS 12 REPS CIRCUIT FOR 6 MINUTES | | | | | |
| | | | | ✓ | |

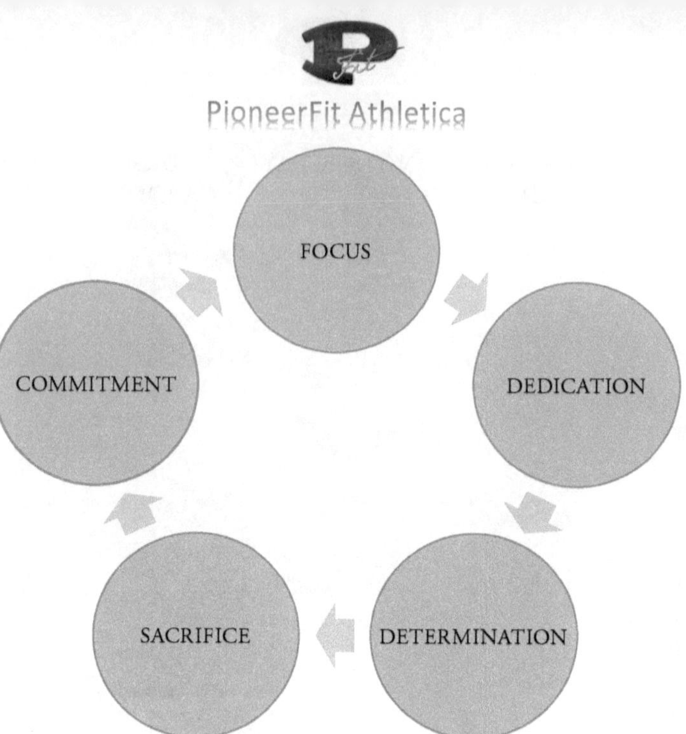

FOCUS
DEDICATION
DETERMINATION
SACRIFICE
COMMITMENT

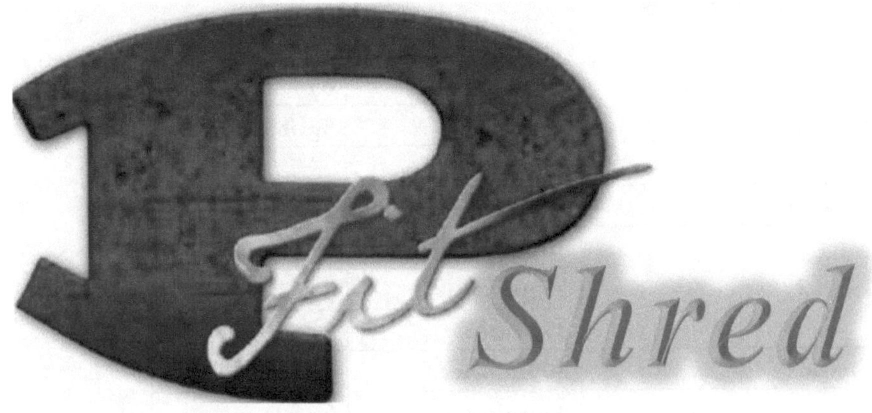


Welcome to the pioneer Fit shred nutrition guide. This is your key to success! Following this meal plan will help you eat right for 4 weeks, 8 weeks or 12 weeks and build lean, strong muscle.

Our program is designed to be simple and easy to follow, this plan outlines daily meals for 8 weeks. Each meal should take 15 minutes or less to prepare.

During weeks 1- 4, you Will clean your system, so you burn fat. You will balance your hormones and get your body properly fueled for weeks 5-8.

Weeks 5-8 will increase and sustain muscle. These weeks include 1 additional meal and 1 additional snack. The post workout meal must be eaten within 20-30 minutes following our pioneer Fit Shred workout and the optional snack is available if you need more energy.

The nutrition plan is not only about dropping fat and increasing muscle but choosing foods that are nutrient dense for optimal health. The foods in this meal plan will help increase your energy, athletic performance, speed and strength.

Each major meal contains a lean source of high energy protein. Protein will aid in sustained energy and keeping hormone levels balanced. Within 2 weeks of adopting this plan, you should feel the difference of healthy, well-balanced meals!

## EXAMPLE PLAN

| | | |
|---|---|---|
| Meal 1 | 300calories | 6g fat |
| | 25gprotein | 5gfiber |
| | 34gcarbs | |
| Snack 1 | 150calories | 4g fat |
| Meal 2 | 300calories | 6g fat |
| | 25gprotein | 5g fiber |
| | 25g carbs | |
| Snack 2 | 200calories | 4g fat |
| Meal 3 | 350calories | 6g fat |
| | 25gprotein | 5g fiber |
| | 25g carbs | |
| Snack optional | 180calories | 4g fat |
| Post workout meal | 180calories | 4g fat |

## HERE ARE YOUR WEEKLY MEAL PLANS TO HELP YOU KICK START YOUR FAT BURN.

### Week 1 Day 1

| Meal 1 – Oatmeal | | |
|---|---|---|
| 2/3 cup oatmeal (non-instant) | | 2tsp. maple syrup or natural sweetener |
| | Side | ½ cup of milk or yogurt |
| | Drink | Water |
| Snack 1 | | 6 Oz. light Greek yogurt |
| | Drink | Water |
| Meal 2 – soup and salad | | |
| 1 ½ cups broth-based soup | | 2 cups tossed greens with vegetables |
| ¼ cup cottage cheese or non-fat dressing | | |
| | Drink | Water |
| Snack 2 | | Protein bar, no more than 220 calories and 5g of fat. |
| | Drink | Water |

| Meal 3 – Lemon and Ginger Salmon | |
|---|---|
| 6 oz salmon | Lemon and fresh ginger |
| Top salmon with lemon and fresh ginger and fold tightly in tinfoil. Bake at 350 for about 20-25 minutes. | |

| | Side | 1 cup steamed vegetables 1cup quinoa |
|---|---|---|
| | Drink | Water |

## Week 1 Day 2

| Meal 1 – Cereal | | |
|---|---|---|
| 1 cup non-sweetened whole grain cereal<br>1 cup water | | 1 cup of low fat milk |
| | Side | 1 serving of fruit |
| | Drink | Water |
| Snack 1 | | 10 – 15 baby carrots -2 tbsp low fat ranch dressing |
| | Drink | Water |
| Meal 2 – whole wheat sandwich | | |
| 2 slices whole wheat or Ezekiel bread | | 1 tbsp. light miracle whip or light mayo/mustard |
| 4 slices lean turkey or another lean deli meat | | Tomato, lettuce, or others to taste |
| | Drink | Water |
| Snack 2 | | 1 banana, 1 handful of nuts |
| | Drink | Water |
| Meal 3 – feta chicken salad | | |
| 6 oz cooked chicken breast, sliced | | Feta cheese, shredded lettuce |
| Shredded lettuce with cooked chicken. Sprinkled with feta cheese | | |
| | Side | 1 serving of fruit |
| | Drink | Water |

## Week 1 Day 3

| Meal 1 – Blueberry Oat Pancakes | |
|---|---|
| 1 cup old fashioned oats | 2 large eggs |
| 1 cup blueberries | 1 tsp. vanilla extract |

| ½ cup low-fat cottage cheese | 1 tsp. 100% maple syrup or 2/3 cup of light reek yogurt. |
|---|---|
| In a blender, combine oats, cottage cheese, eggs and vanilla extract. Stir in blueberries. Scoop batter onto warm skillet and make 3-4inch pancakes. Cook until brown on each side. Top with maple syrup or Greek yogurt. | |

| | Drink | Water |
|---|---|---|
| Snack 1 | | 1 serving of fruit -1 string cheese |
| | Drink | Water |

| Meal 2 – grilled chicken | |
|---|---|
| 6oz chicken breast | 2 cups tossed greens with vegetables |
| Top chicken breast with your favorite herbs and spices. Bake at 350 for 20-30 minutes or grill tor approximately 20 minutes. | |
| 4 cups tossed greens with vegetables ½ cup cottage cheese | |

| | Drink | Water |
|---|---|---|
| Snack 2 | | ¼ cup cottage cheese- 1 serving of fruit |
| | Drink | Water |

| Meal 3 – stir fry | |
|---|---|
| 1 cup cooked rice | 1 ½ cups vegetables |
| 1 cup light coconut milk | Curry spice to taste |
| Place vegetables in saucepan. Add milk and curry spice. Cook until vegetables are done then place mixture on top of cooked rice. | |

| | Drink | Water |
|---|---|---|

## Week 1 Day 4

| Meal 1 – shake and oatmeal | |
|---|---|
| 1 scoop of whey protein | ½ cup skim, almond, or rice milk |
| 1 whole banana | Ice |
| ½ cup of water | 2/3 cup oatmeal 2tsp maple syrup |

| | Side | ½ cup of milk or yogurt |
|---|---|---|
| | Drink | Water |
| Snack 1 | | ½ cup low-fat cottage cheese – 1 cup fruit |
| | Drink | Water |

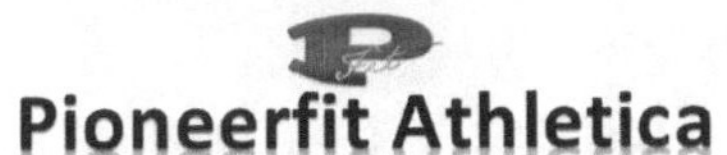

# Pioneerfit Athletica

| Meal 2 – turkey pita | |
| --- | --- |
| 1 large wheat pita | 1 tbsp. light miracle whip or light mayonnaise |
| 4 slices lean turkey or another lean deli meat | ½ tbsp. mustard |
| 1 oz. slice of cheese | Tomato, cucumber, lettuce, sprouts, other vegetables |
| Spread miracle whip and mustard on the pita. Fill pita with meat, cheese and vegetables. | |

| | side | 4 celery sticks, 1 cup raw broccoli, 2 tbsp. low-fat dressing |
| --- | --- | --- |
| | drink | Water |
| Snack 2 | | 1 serving of fruit<br>1 part-skim mozzarella string cheese |
| | Drink | Water |

| Meal 3 – grilled teriyaki tuna | |
| --- | --- |
| 4 oz. tuna steak | 1/3 cup cooked brown rice |
| 2 tbsp. low-fat, bottled teriyaki sauce | Fresh spinach 1 tsp. olive oil |
| Place tuna steak in saucepan with olive oil. Cook approximately 10 minutes or until meat is done. Add teriyaki sauce and place on top of rice with a side of fresh spinach. | |

| | Drink | Water |
| --- | --- | --- |

## Week 1 Day 5

| Meal 1 – veggie egg white omelet | |
| --- | --- |
| 4 – 5 egg whites | 1 plum tomato, chopped |
| 1 egg yolk | 1 small clove of garlic, chopped |
| 2 tbsp. skim milk | 1 handful spinach, shredded |
| 1 tbsp. onion, minced | Lite cooking spray |
| Place eggs, milk, vegetables and garlic in bowl or blender and mix together. Spray large skillet with cooking spray and place mixture in pan. Cook on both sides until done. | |

| | Drink | Water |
| --- | --- | --- |
| Snack 1 | | 1 cup grapes – ¼ cup almonds |
| | Drink | Water |

| Meal 2 – Avocado and chicken salad | | |
|---|---|---|
| 4 oz. grilled chicken | | ½ cup orange, sliced |
| 3 cup mixed greens | | 1 tbsp. lemon juice |
| ¼ cup avocado, sliced | | 2 tsp. olive oil |
| Top mixed greens with orange, avocado and chicken. Drizzle with olive oil and lemon juice. | | |
| | Drink | Water |
| Snack 2 | | 10 – 15 baby carrots- 2tbsp. low-fat ranch dip |
| | Drink | Water |
| Meal 3 – BLT with Turkey | | |
| 2 slices whole wheat bread | | Tomato, sliced |
| 3 slices turkey bacon | | Lettuce, to taste |
| | Sides | 1 serving of fruit |
| | Drink | water |

# Week 1 Day 6

| Meal 1 – Blueberry Oat Pancakes | | |
|---|---|---|
| 1 cup old fashioned oats | | 2 large eggs |
| 1 cup blueberries | | 1 tsp. vanilla extract |
| ½ cup low-fat cottage cheese | | 1 tsp. 100% maple syrup or 2/3 cup of light reek yogurt. |
| In a blender, combine oats, cottage cheese, eggs and vanilla extract. Stir in blueberries. Scoop batter onto warm skillet and make 3-4inch pancakes. Cook until brown on each side. Top with maple syrup or Greek yogurt. | | |
| | Drink | Water |
| Snack 1 | | 1 serving of fruit -1 string cheese |
| | Drink | Water |
| Meal 2 – minestrone soup | | |
| 1 ½ cups low sodium minestrone soup | | 1 whole grain roll or toast |
| | Side | 1 tomato, sliced 1 oz. mozzarella, sliced basil and balsamic vinegar |
| | Drink | Water |
| Snack 2 | | 1 cup grapes – ¼ cup almonds |
| | Drink | Water |

| Meal 3 – Roast beef pita | |
| --- | --- |
| 4 oz. lean roast beef or other lean meat | Dark salad greens |
| 3 – inch whole wheat pita | Bell peppers, sliced |
| Cherry tomatoes, sliced | Cucumbers, sliced |
| Romaine lettuce | Mushrooms, sliced |
| | Drink | Water |

## Week 1 Day 7

| Meal 1 – egg burrito | | |
| --- | --- | --- |
| 4 small whole grain tortillas | | ½ cup sweet onion, chopped |
| 2 cups egg white | | Salt and pepper |
| ½ cup low-fat cottage cheese | | ½ cup black beans |
| ½ cup tomatoes, chopped | | Lite cooking spray |
| ½ cup red or green sweet pepper, chopped | | |
| Spray large skillet with cooking spray. Add eggs, cottage cheese, vegetables and beans. Stir together. Once fully cooked, place mixture on tortillas. Salt and pepper to taste. | | |
| | side | ½ cup milk or yogurt |
| | Drink | Water |
| Snack 1 | | 2 slices turkey jerky |
| | Drink | Water |
| Meal 2 – Meatballs and Marinara | | |
| 4oz. extra-lean ground turkey | | 2 tbsp. parmesan cheese, grated |
| ½ cup marinara sauce | | Lite cooking spray |
| Roll ground turkey into 3-4 balls. Spray pan with cooking spray and cook meatballs approximately 7 minutes. Top meatballs with marinara sauce and parmesan cheese. | | |
| | Drink | Water |
| Snack 2 | | 6 oz. light Greek yogurt |
| | Drink | Water |
| Meal 3 – bagel sandwich | | |
| ½ whole wheat bagel or 1 slice toast | | 1 slice reduced fat cheese |
| 2 oz. deli style turkey breast, sliced | | Tomato, sliced |
| | Drink | Water |

## Week 2 day 1

| Meal 1 – oatmeal | | |
| --- | --- | --- |
| 2/3 cup old fashioned oats | | 2 tsp. 100% maple syrup or natural sweetener |
| 1 cup water | | |
| Follow oatmeal instructions and top with maple syrup. | | |
| | Side | ½ cup milk or yogurt |
| | Drink | Water |
| Snack 1 | | 6oz light Greek yogurt or kefir |
| | Drink | Water |
| Meal 2 – peanut butter and banana | | |
| 1 slice whole grain or Ezekiel bread | | 1 tbsp. all fruit preserves or banana |
| 1 tbsp. natural peanut butter | | |
| | Drink | Water |
| Snack 2 | | Protein bar, no more than 220 calories and 5 g of fat |
| | Drink | Water |
| Meal 3 – turkey burger | | |
| 4oz. lean ground turkey | | 2 tbsp. red onion, chopped |
| 2 tbsp. salsa | | 1 whole grain pita |
| Form ground turkey into a patty. Cook turkey approximately 4 minutes on each side until done. Top with salsa and onion and place in whole grain pita. | | |
| | Side | 1 cup steamed vegetables |
| | Drinks | Water |

## Week 2 Day 2

| Meal 1 – cereal | | |
| --- | --- | --- |
| 1 cup non-sweetened whole grain cereal | | 1 cup low-fat milk |
| | Drink | Water |
| Snack 1 | | ½ cup low-fat cottage cheese- 1 serving of fruit. |
| | Drink | Water |
| Meal 2 – grilled chicken salad | | |
| 3oz grilled chicken breast | | 1 tbsp. pecans, chopped |

| | | |
|---|---|---|
| 3 cups mixed dark greens | | Cucumber, sliced |
| ½ apple, chopped | | |
| Top mixed greens with chicken, chopped apple, pecans and cucumber to taste. | | |
| | Drink | Water |
| Snack 2 | | 1 banana- 1 handful nuts |
| | Drink | Water |
| **Meal 3 – marinated turkey** | | |
| 4oz. marinated turkey tenderloins | | ½ cup long grain and wild rice |
| Marinate turkey tenderloin in your favorite sauce for 20 minutes. Bake at 350 for 30 minutes or cook over medium heat for approximately 10 minutes on each side or until done. | | |
| | Side | ½ cup green peas 1 cup fresh fruit. |
| | Drink | Water |

## Week 2 Day 3

| | | |
|---|---|---|
| **Meal 1 – buckwheat cereal** | | |
| 2/3 cup buckwheat cereal | | ½ banana |
| 1 cup water | | 1 tsp. 100% maple syrup |
| Mix buckwheat cereal with water and cook for 20 minutes on the stove, top with banana and syrup. | | |
| | Drink | 1 cup of milk |
| Snack 1 | | 1 serving of fruit -1 mozzarella string cheese |
| | Drink | Water |
| **Meal 2 – grilled chicken wrap** | | |
| 6-inch whole grain tortilla | | Red bell pepper, sliced |
| 3 oz. grilled chicken breast | | Lettuce |
| Tomato, sliced | | |
| | Side | Celery sticks 1 tbsp. low fat ranch dressing |
| | Drink | Water |
| Snack 2 | | ¼ cup cottage cheese- 1 serving of fruit |
| | Drink | Water |
| **Meal 3 – lemon chicken** | | |

| 6 oz. chicken breast | 1 ½ cups vegetables |
|---|---|
| 1 lemon | |
| Squeeze lemon juice over chicken. Bake at 350 for 20-30 minutes. Bake assorted vegetables at 350 for 10-15 minutes. | |

| | Side | ½ cup fresh fruit |
|---|---|---|
| | Drink | Water |

## Week 2 Day4

| Meal 1 – shake | | |
|---|---|---|
| 1 scoop whey protein | | 1 tsp. peanut butter |
| ½ cup fat free milk | | Handful of ice |
| ½ cup water | | |
| | Drink | Water |
| Snack 1 | | 10 -15 baby carrots- 2tbsp. low fat ranch dip |
| | Drink | Water |
| **Meal 2 – turkey pita** | | |
| 1 large wheat pita | | 1 tbsp. light miracle whip or light mayo |
| 4 slices lean turkey | | Tomato, cucumber, lettuce, sprouts or another veg. |
| 1 oz. slice of cheese | | ½ tbsp. mustard |
| Spread miracle whip and mustard on the pita. Fill pita with turkey, cheese and vegetables. | | |
| | Side | 4 celery sticks 1 cup raw broccoli 2 tbsp. low fat dressing |
| | Drink | Water |
| Snack 2 | | 1 serving of fruit – 1-part skim mozzarella string cheese |
| | Drink | Water |
| **Meal 3 – meaty turkey burger 1 burger per serving** | | |
| 1 lb. extra lean ground turkey | | ¼ cup low fat chicken or vegetable stock |
| ½ cup oat bran | | 1 clove of garlic, pressed |
| 2 tbsp. flaxseed | | 1 tbsp. soy sauce |
| 2 egg whites | | 1 whole wheat bun |

Mix ground turkey with oat bran, flaxseed, egg whites, stock, garlic and soy sauce. Form into 3 patties and cook approximately 5 minutes on each side or until done. Place on whole wheat bun.

| | |
|---|---|
| Side | 1 cup steamed vegetables |
| Drink | Water |

## Week 2 Day 5

| Meal 1 – veggie egg white omelet | |
|---|---|
| 4-5 egg whites | 1 plum tomato, chopped |
| 1 egg yolk | 1 small clove of garlic, chopped |
| 2 tbsp. skim milk | 1 handful spinach, shredded |
| 1 tbsp. onion, minced | Lite cooking spray |

Place eggs, milk, vegetables and garlic in bowl or blender and mix together. Spray large skillet with cooking spray and place mixture in pan. Cook on both sides until done.

| | |
|---|---|
| Drink | Water |
| Snack 1 | 1 cup grapes- ¼ cup almonds |
| Drink | Water |

| Meal 2 – avocado and chicken salad | |
|---|---|
| 4 oz. grilled chicken | ½ cup orange, sliced |
| 3 cups mixed greens | 1 tbsp. lemon juice |
| ¼ cup avocado, sliced | 2 tsp. olive oil |

Top mixed greens with orange, avocado and chicken. Drizzle with olive oil and lemon juice. breast with your favorite herbs and spices.

| | |
|---|---|
| Drink | Water |
| Snack 2 | ¼ cup cottage cheese- 1 serving of fruit |
| Drink | Water |

| Meal 3 – black bean soup and sandwich | |
|---|---|
| 1 cup of canned black bean soup | 2 thin sliced avocados |
| 1 slice whole grain bread | 1 tsp. Dijon mustard |
| 2 oz. deli style turkey breast, sliced | |

Spread Dijon mustard over bread. Top with turkey and avocado

| | |
|---|---|
| Drink | Water |

## Week 2 Day 6

| Meal 1 – Blueberry Oat Pancakes | |
|---|---|
| 1 cup old fashioned oats | 2 large eggs |
| 1 cup blueberries | 1 tsp. vanilla extract |
| ½ cup low-fat cottage cheese | 1 tsp. 100% maple syrup or 2/3 cup of light reek yogurt. |
| In a blender, combine oats, cottage cheese, eggs and vanilla extract. Stir in blueberries. Scoop batter onto warm skillet and make 3-4-inch pancakes. Cook until brown on each side. Top with maple syrup or Greek yogurt. | |
| Drink | Water |
| Snack 1 | 1 serving of fruit -1 string cheese |
| Drink | Water |
| Meal 2 – grilled chicken | |
| 6oz chicken breast | 2 cups tossed greens with vegetables |
| Top chicken breast with your favorite herbs and spices. Bake at 350 for 20-30 minutes or grill tor approximately 20 minutes. | |
| 4 cups tossed greens with vegetables ½ cup cottage cheese | |
| Drink | Water |
| Snack 2 | ¼ cup cottage cheese- 1 serving of fruit |
| Drink | Water |
| Meal 3 – stir fry | |
| 1 cup cooked rice | 1 ½ cups vegetables |
| 1 cup light coconut milk | Curry spice to taste |
| Place vegetables in saucepan. Add milk and curry spice. Cook until vegetables are done then place mixture on top of cooked rice. | |
| Drink | Water |

## Week 2 Day 7

| Meal 1 – egg burrito | |
|---|---|
| 4 small whole grain tortillas | ½ cup sweet onion, chopped |
| 2 cups egg whites | ½ cup black beans |
| ½ cup low-fat cottage cheese | Salt and pepper |
| ½ cup tomatoes, chopped | Lite cooking spray |

| | | |
|---|---|---|
| ½ cup red or green sweet pepper, chopped. | | |
| Spray large skillet with cooking spray. Add eggs, cottage cheese, vegetables and beans. Stir together. Once fully cooked, place mixture on tortillas. Salt and pepper to taste. | | |
| | Drink | Water |
| Snack 1 | | 2 slices of turkey jerky |
| | Drink | Water |
| **Meal 2 – meatballs and marinara** | | |
| 4 oz. extra lean | | 2 tbsp. parmesan cheese, grated |
| ½ cup marinara sauce | | Lite cooking spray |
| Roll ground turkey into 3 -4 balls. Spray pan with cooking spray and cook meatballs approximately 7 minutes. Top meatballs with marinara sauce and parmesan cheese. | | |
| | Drink | Water |
| Snack 2 | | 6 oz. light Greek yogurt |
| | Drink | Water |
| **Meal 3 – rosemary chicken** | | |
| 4 oz chicken | | 2 cups arugula |
| 1tsp. rosemary | | 1tbsp. parmesan cheese grated |
| ½ tsp. garlic, minced | | 1 tsp. olive oil |
| Top chicken with rosemary, garlic and olive oil. Wrap in tin foil and bake at 350 for 20 minutes or until fully cooked. Top arugula with the chicken and sprinkle with parmesan cheese. | | |
| | Side | 1 cup of beets |
| | Drink | Water |

## Week 3 Day 1

| **Meal 1 – Blueberry Oat Pancakes** | |
|---|---|
| 1 cup old fashioned oats | 2 large eggs |
| 1 cup blueberries | 1 tsp. vanilla extract |
| ½ cup low-fat cottage cheese | 1 tsp. 100% maple syrup or 2/3 cup of light reek yogurt. |

| | | |
|---|---|---|
| In a blender, combine oats, cottage cheese, eggs and vanilla extract. Stir in blueberries. Scoop batter onto warm skillet and make 3-4inch pancakes. Cook until brown on each side. Top with maple syrup or Greek yogurt. | | |
| | Drink | Water |
| Snack 1 | | 1 serving of fruit -1 string cheese |
| | Drink | Water |
| **Meal 2 – grilled chicken** | | |
| 6oz chicken breast | | 2 cups tossed greens with vegetables |
| Top chicken breast with your favorite herbs and spices. Bake at 350 for 20-30 minutes or grill tor approximately 20 minutes. | | |
| 4 cups tossed greens with vegetables ½ cup cottage cheese | | |
| | Drink | Water |
| Snack 2 | | ¼ cup cottage cheese- 1 serving of fruit |
| | Drink | Water |
| **Meal 3 – stir fry** | | |
| 1 cup cooked rice | | 1 ½ cups vegetables |
| 1 cup light coconut milk | | Curry spice to taste |
| Place vegetables in saucepan. Add milk and curry spice. Cook until vegetables are done then place mixture on top of cooked rice. | | |
| | Drink | Water |

## Week 3 Day 2

| | | |
|---|---|---|
| **Meal 1 – Oatmeal** | | |
| 2/3 cup oatmeal (non-instant) | | 2tsp. maple syrup or natural sweetener |
| | Side | ½ cup of milk or yogurt |
| | Drink | Water |
| Snack 1 | | 6 0z. light Greek yogurt |
| | Drink | Water |
| **Meal 2 – soup and salad** | | |
| 1 ½ cups broth-based soup | | 2 cups tossed greens with vegetables |
| ¼ cup cottage cheese or non-fat dressing | | |
| | Drink | Water |

# Pioneerfit Athletica

| Snack 2 | | Protein bar, no more than 220 calories and 5g of fat. |
|---|---|---|
| | Drink | Water |
| **Meal 3 – Lemon and Ginger Salmon** | | |
| 6 oz salmon | | Lemon and fresh ginger |
| Top salmon with lemon and fresh ginger and fold tightly in tinfoil. Bake at 350 for about 20-25 minutes. | | |
| | Side | 1 cup steamed vegetables 1cup quinoa |
| | Drink | Water |

## Week 3 Day 3

| **Meal 1 – Cereal** | | |
|---|---|---|
| 1 cup non-sweetened whole grain cereal<br>1 cup water | | 1 cup of low fat milk |
| | Side | 1 serving of fruit |
| | Drink | Water |
| Snack 1 | | 10 – 15 baby carrots -2 tbsp low fat ranch dressing |
| | Drink | Water |
| **Meal 2 – whole wheat sandwich** | | |
| 2 slices whole wheat or Ezekiel bread | | 1 tbsp. light miracle whip or light mayo/mustard |
| 4 slices lean turkey or another lean deli meat | | Tomato, lettuce, or others to taste |
| | Drink | Water |
| Snack 2 | | 1 banana, 1 handful of nuts |
| | Drink | Water |
| **Meal 3 – feta chicken salad** | | |
| 6 oz cooked chicken breast, sliced | | Feta cheese, shredded lettuce |
| Shredded lettuce with cooked chicken. Sprinkled with feta cheese | | |
| | Side | 1 serving of fruit |
| | Drink | Water |

## Week 3 Day 4

| Meal 1 – Blueberry Oat Pancakes | |
|---|---|
| 1 cup old fashioned oats | 2 large eggs |
| 1 cup blueberries | 1 tsp. vanilla extract |
| ½ cup low-fat cottage cheese | 1 tsp. 100% maple syrup or 2/3 cup of light reek yogurt. |
| In a blender, combine oats, cottage cheese, eggs and vanilla extract. Stir in blueberries. Scoop batter onto warm skillet and make 3-4-inch pancakes. Cook until brown on each side. Top with maple syrup or Greek yogurt. | |
| Drink | Water |
| Snack 1 | 1 serving of fruit -1 string cheese |
| Drink | Water |
| Meal 2 – grilled chicken | |
| 6oz chicken breast | 2 cups tossed greens with vegetables |
| Top chicken breast with your favorite herbs and spices. Bake at 350 for 20-30 minutes or grill tor approximately 20 minutes. | |
| 4 cups tossed greens with vegetables ½ cup cottage cheese | |
| Drink | Water |
| Snack 2 | ¼ cup cottage cheese- 1 serving of fruit |
| Drink | Water |
| Meal 3 – stir fry | |
| 1 cup cooked rice | 1 ½ cups vegetables |
| 1 cup light coconut milk | Curry spice to taste |
| Place vegetables in saucepan. Add milk and curry spice. Cook until vegetables are done then place mixture on top of cooked rice. | |
| Drink | Water |

## Week 3 Day5

| Meal 1 – veggie egg white omelet | |
|---|---|
| 4 – 5 egg whites | 1 plum tomato, chopped |
| 1 egg yolk | 1 small clove of garlic, chopped |
| 2 tbsp. skim milk | 1 handful spinach, shredded |
| 1 tbsp. onion, minced | Lite cooking spray |

# Pioneerfit Athletica

| | | |
|---|---|---|
| Place eggs, milk, vegetables and garlic in bowl or blender and mix together. Spray large skillet with cooking spray and place mixture in pan. Cook on both sides until done. | | |
| | Drink | Water |
| Snack 1 | | 1 cup grapes – ¼ cup almonds |
| | Drink | Water |
| **Meal 2 – Avocado and chicken salad** | | |
| 4 oz. grilled chicken | | ½ cup orange, sliced |
| 3 cup mixed greens | | 1 tbsp. lemon juice |
| ¼ cup avocado, sliced | | 2 tsp. olive oil |
| Top mixed greens with orange, avocado and chicken. Drizzle with olive oil and lemon juice. | | |
| | Drink | Water |
| Snack 2 | | 10 – 15 baby carrots- 2tbsp. low-fat ranch dip |
| | Drink | Water |
| **Meal 3 – BLT with Turkey** | | |
| 2 slices whole wheat bread | | Tomato, sliced |
| 3 slices turkey bacon | | Lettuce, to taste |
| | Sides | 1 serving of fruit |
| | Drink | water |

## Week 3 Day 6

| | | |
|---|---|---|
| **Meal 1 – Blueberry Oat Pancakes** | | |
| 1 cup old fashioned oats | | 2 large eggs |
| 1 cup blueberries | | 1 tsp. vanilla extract |
| ½ cup low-fat cottage cheese | | 1 tsp. 100% maple syrup or 2/3 cup of light reek yogurt. |
| In a blender, combine oats, cottage cheese, eggs and vanilla extract. Stir in blueberries. Scoop batter onto warm skillet and make 3-4-inch pancakes. Cook until brown on each side. Top with maple syrup or Greek yogurt. | | |
| | Drink | Water |
| Snack 1 | | 1 serving of fruit -1 string cheese |
| | Drink | Water |

| Meal 2 – minestrone soup | | |
|---|---|---|
| 1 ½ cups low sodium minestrone soup | | 1 whole grain roll or toast |
| | Side | 1 tomato, sliced 1 oz. mozzarella, sliced basil and balsamic vinegar |
| | Drink | Water |
| Snack 2 | | 1 cup grapes – ¼ cup almonds |
| | Drink | Water |
| Meal 3 – Roast beef pita | | |
| 4 oz. lean roast beef or other lean meat | | Dark salad greens |
| 3 – inch whole wheat pita | | Bell peppers, sliced |
| Cherry tomatoes, sliced | | Cucumbers, sliced |
| Romaine lettuce | | Mushrooms, sliced |
| | Drink | Water |

## Week 3 Day 7

| Meal 1 – egg burrito | |
|---|---|
| 4 small whole grain tortillas | ½ cup sweet onion, chopped |
| 2 cups egg white | Salt and pepper |
| ½ cup low-fat cottage cheese | ½ cup black beans |
| ½ cup tomatoes, chopped | Lite cooking spray |
| ½ cup red or green sweet pepper, chopped | |

Spray large skillet with cooking spray. Add eggs, cottage cheese, vegetables and beans. Stir together. Once fully cooked, place mixture on tortillas. Salt and pepper to taste.

| | Side | ½ cup milk or yogurt |
|---|---|---|
| | Drink | Water |
| Snack 1 | | 2 slices turkey jerky |
| | Drink | Water |
| Meal 2 – Meatballs and Marinara | | |
| 4oz. extra-lean ground turkey | | 2 tbsp. parmesan cheese, grated |
| ½ cup marinara sauce | | Lite cooking spray |

| | | |
|---|---|---|
| Roll ground turkey into 3-4 balls. Spray pan with cooking spray and cook meatballs approximately 7 minutes. Top meatballs with marinara sauce and parmesan cheese. | | |
| | Drink | Water |
| Snack 2 | | 6 oz. light Greek yogurt |
| | Drink | Water |
| **Meal 3 – bagel sandwich** | | |
| ½ whole wheat bagel or 1 slice toast | | 1 slice reduced fat cheese |
| 2 oz. deli style turkey breast, sliced | | Tomato, sliced |
| | Drink | Water |

## Week 4 day 1

| | | |
|---|---|---|
| **Meal 1 – oatmeal** | | |
| 2/3 cup old fashioned oats | | 2 tsp. 100% maple syrup or natural sweetener |
| 1 cup water | | |
| Follow oatmeal instructions and top with maple syrup. | | |
| | Side | ½ cup milk or yogurt |
| | Drink | Water |
| Snack 1 | | 6oz light Greek yogurt or kefir |
| | Drink | Water |
| **Meal 2 – peanut butter and banana** | | |
| 1 slice whole grain or Ezekiel bread | | 1 tbsp. all fruit preserves or banana |
| 1 tbsp. natural peanut butter | | |
| | Drink | Water |
| Snack 2 | | Protein bar, no more than 220 calories and 5 g of fat |
| | Drink | Water |
| **Meal 3 – turkey burger** | | |
| 4oz. lean ground turkey | | 2 tbsp. red onion, chopped |
| 2 tbsp. salsa | | 1 whole grain pita |
| Form ground turkey into a patty. Cook turkey approximately 4 minutes on each side until done. Top with salsa and onion and place in whole grain pita. | | |

| Side | 1 cup steamed vegetables |
|---|---|
| Drinks | Water |

## Week 4 day 2

| Meal 1 – cereal | |
|---|---|
| 1 cup non-sweetened whole grain cereal | 1 cup low-fat milk |
| Drink | Water |
| Snack 1 | ½ cup low-fat cottage cheese- 1 serving of fruit. |
| Drink | Water |

| Meal 2 – grilled chicken salad | |
|---|---|
| 3oz grilled chicken breast | 1 tbsp. pecans, chopped |
| 3 cups mixed dark greens | Cucumber, sliced |
| ½ apple, chopped | |
| Top mixed greens with chicken, chopped apple, pecans and cucumber to taste. | |
| Drink | Water |
| Snack 2 | 1 banana- 1 handful nuts |
| Drink | Water |

| Meal 3 – marinated turkey | |
|---|---|
| 4oz. marinated turkey tenderloins | ½ cup long grain and wild rice |
| Marinate turkey tenderloin in your favorite sauce for 20 minutes. Bake at 350 for 30 minutes or cook over medium heat for approximately 10 minutes on each side or until done. | |
| Side | ½ cup green peas 1 cup fresh fruit. |
| Drink | Water |

## Week 4 day 3

| Meal 1 – buckwheat cereal | |
|---|---|
| 2/3 cup buckwheat cereal | ½ banana |
| 1 cup water | 1 tsp. 100% maple syrup |
| Mix buckwheat cereal with water and cook for 20 minutes on the stove, top with banana and syrup. | |

|  | Drink | 1 cup of milk |
|---|---|---|
| Snack 1 |  | 1 serving of fruit -1 mozzarella string cheese |
|  | Drink | Water |
| **Meal 2 – grilled chicken wrap** | | |
| 6-inch whole grain tortilla |  | Red bell pepper, sliced |
| 3 oz. grilled chicken breast |  | Lettuce |
| Tomato, sliced |  |  |
|  | Side | Celery sticks 1 tbsp. low fat ranch dressing |
|  | Drink | Water |
| Snack 2 |  | ¼ cup cottage cheese- 1 serving of fruit |
|  | Drink | Water |
| **Meal 3 – lemon chicken** | | |
| 6 oz. chicken breast |  | 1 ½ cups vegetables |
| 1 lemon |  |  |
| Squeeze lemon juice over chicken. Bake at 350 for 20-30 minutes. Bake assorted vegetables at 350 for 10-15 minutes. | | |
|  | Side | ½ cup fresh fruit |
|  | Drink | Water |

## Week 4 day 4

| **Meal 1 – shake** | | |
|---|---|---|
| 1 scoop whey protein |  | 1 tsp. peanut butter |
| ½ cup fat free milk |  | Handful of ice |
| ½ cup water |  |  |
|  | Drink | Water |
| Snack 1 |  | 10 -15 baby carrots- 2tbsp. low fat ranch dip |
|  | Drink | Water |
| **Meal 2 – turkey pita** | | |
| 1 large wheat pita |  | 1 tbsp. light miracle whip or light mayo |

# Pioneerfit Athletica

| | | |
|---|---|---|
| 4 slices lean turkey | | Tomato, cucumber, lettuce, sprouts or another veg. |
| 1 oz. slice of cheese | | ½ tbsp. mustard |
| Spread miracle whip and mustard on the pita. Fill pita with turkey, cheese and vegetables. | | |
| | Side | 4 celery sticks 1 cup raw broccoli 2 tbsp. low fat dressing |
| | Drink | Water |
| Snack 2 | | 1 serving of fruit – 1-part skim mozzarella string cheese |
| | Drink | Water |

| Meal 3 – meaty turkey burger 1 burger per serving | | |
|---|---|---|
| 1 lb. extra lean ground turkey | | ¼ cup low fat chicken or vegetable stock |
| ½ cup oat bran | | 1 clove of garlic, pressed |
| 2 tbsp. flaxseed | | 1 tbsp. soy sauce |
| 2 egg whites | | 1 whole wheat bun |
| Mix ground turkey with oat bran, flaxseed, egg whites, stock, garlic and soy sauce. Form into 3 patties and cook approximately 5 minutes on each side or until done. Place on whole wheat bun. | | |
| | Side | 1 cup steamed vegetables |
| | Drink | Water |

## Week 4 day 5

| Meal 1 – veggie egg white omelet | | |
|---|---|---|
| 4-5 egg whites | | 1 plum tomato, chopped |
| 1 egg yolk | | 1 small clove of garlic, chopped |
| 2 tbsp. skim milk | | 1 handful spinach, shredded |
| 1 tbsp. onion, minced | | Lite cooking spray |
| Place eggs, milk, vegetables and garlic in bowl or blender and mix together. Spray large skillet with cooking spray and place mixture in pan. Cook on both sides until done. | | |
| | Drink | Water |
| Snack 1 | | 1 cup grapes- ¼ cup almonds |
| | Drink | Water |

| Meal 2 – avocado and chicken salad | |
| --- | --- |
| 4 oz. grilled chicken | ½ cup orange, sliced |
| 3 cups mixed greens | 1 tbsp. lemon juice |
| ¼ cup avocado, sliced | 2 tsp. olive oil |
| Top mixed greens with orange, avocado and chicken. Drizzle with olive oil and lemon juice. breast with your favorite herbs and spices. | |

| | Drink | Water |
| --- | --- | --- |
| Snack 2 | | ¼ cup cottage cheese- 1 serving of fruit |
| | Drink | Water |

| Meal 3 – black bean soup and sandwich | |
| --- | --- |
| 1 cup of canned black bean soup | 2 thin sliced avocados |
| 1 slice whole grain bread | 1 tsp. Dijon mustard |
| 2 oz. deli style turkey breast, sliced | |
| Spread Dijon mustard over bread. Top with turkey and avocado | |

| | Drink | Water |
| --- | --- | --- |

# Week 4 day 6

| Meal 1 – Blueberry Oat Pancakes | |
| --- | --- |
| 1 cup old fashioned oats | 2 large eggs |
| 1 cup blueberries | 1 tsp. vanilla extract |
| ½ cup low-fat cottage cheese | 1 tsp. 100% maple syrup or 2/3 cup of light reek yogurt. |
| In a blender, combine oats, cottage cheese, eggs and vanilla extract. Stir in blueberries. Scoop batter onto warm skillet and make 3-4-inch pancakes. Cook until brown on each side. Top with maple syrup or Greek yogurt. | |

| | Drink | Water |
| --- | --- | --- |
| Snack 1 | | 1 serving of fruit -1 string cheese |
| | Drink | Water |

| Meal 2 – grilled chicken | |
| --- | --- |
| 6oz chicken breast | 2 cups tossed greens with vegetables |
| Top chicken breast with your favorite herbs and spices. Bake at 350 for 20-30 minutes or grill tor approximately 20 minutes. | |
| 4 cups tossed greens with vegetables ½ cup cottage cheese | |

| | Drink | Water |
| --- | --- | --- |

| Snack 2 | | ¼ cup cottage cheese- 1 serving of fruit |
| --- | --- | --- |
| | Drink | Water |

| Meal 3 – stir fry | | |
| --- | --- | --- |
| 1 cup cooked rice | | 1 ½ cups vegetables |
| 1 cup light coconut milk | | Curry spice to taste |
| Place vegetables in saucepan. Add milk and curry spice. Cook until vegetables are done then place mixture on top of cooked rice. | | |
| | Drink | Water |

## Week 4 day 7

| Meal 1 – egg burrito | | |
| --- | --- | --- |
| 4 small whole grain tortillas | | ½ cup sweet onion, chopped |
| 2 cups egg whites | | ½ cup black beans |
| ½ cup low-fat cottage cheese | | Salt and pepper |
| ½ cup tomatoes, chopped | | Lite cooking spray |
| ½ cup red or green sweet pepper, chopped. | | |
| Spray large skillet with cooking spray. Add eggs, cottage cheese, vegetables and beans. Stir together. Once fully cooked, place mixture on tortillas. Salt and pepper to taste. | | |
| | Drink | Water |
| Snack 1 | | 2 slices of turkey jerky |
| | Drink | Water |

| Meal 2 – meatballs and marinara | | |
| --- | --- | --- |
| 4 oz. extra lean | | 2 tbsp. parmesan cheese, grated |
| ½ cup marinara sauce | | Lite cooking spray |
| Roll ground turkey into 3 -4 balls. Spray pan with cooking spray and cook meatballs approximately 7 minutes. Top meatballs with marinara sauce and parmesan cheese. | | |
| | Drink | Water |
| Snack 2 | | 6 oz. light Greek yogurt |
| | Drink | Water |

| Meal 3 – rosemary chicken | | |
| --- | --- | --- |
| 4 oz chicken | | 2 cups arugula |

| 1tsp. rosemary | 1tbsp. parmesan cheese grated |
| --- | --- |
| ½ tsp. garlic, minced | 1 tsp. olive oil |
| Top chicken with rosemary, garlic and olive oil. Wrap in tin foil and bake at 350 for 20 minutes or until fully cooked. Top arugula with the chicken and sprinkle with parmesan cheese. | |
| | Side | 1 cup of beets |
| | Drink | Water |

## Week 5 day 1

| Meal 1 – oatmeal | | |
| --- | --- | --- |
| 2/3 cup old fashioned oats | | 2 tsp. 100% maple syrup or natural sweetener |
| 1 cup water | | |
| Follow oatmeal instructions and top with maple syrup. | | |
| | Side | ½ cup milk or yogurt |
| | Drink | Water |
| Snack 1 | | 6oz light Greek yogurt or kefir |
| | Drink | Water |
| Meal 2 – peanut butter and banana | | |
| 1 slice whole grain or Ezekiel bread | | 1 tbsp. all fruit preserves or banana |
| 1 tbsp. natural peanut butter | | |
| | Drink | Water |
| Snack 2 | | Protein bar, no more than 220 calories and 5 g of fat |
| | Drink | Water |
| Meal 3 – turkey burger | | |
| 4oz. lean ground turkey | | 2 tbsp. red onion, chopped |
| 2 tbsp. salsa | | 1 whole grain pita |
| Form ground turkey into a patty. Cook turkey approximately 4 minutes on each side until done. Top with salsa and onion and place in whole grain pita. | | |
| | Side | 1 cup steamed vegetables |
| | Drinks | Water |

## Week 5 Day 2

| Meal 1 – turkey bacon on toast | | |
|---|---|---|
| 3 slices of turkey bacon | | 1 slice Ezekiel bread, toasted |
| ½ tomato, sliced | | |
| | Drink | Water |
| Snack 1 | | 10 raw almonds |
| | Drink | Water |
| Pesto spaghetti 1 ½ cup per serving | | |
| 1lb. buckwheat or rice noodles | | ½ cup almonds, chopped |
| 3 quarts water | | ¾ cup parsley |
| 1 tsp. salt | | 2 cloves of garlic, chopped |
| 3 cups fresh basil leaves | | Extra virgin olive oil |
| Boil noodles in water and salt approximately 12 minutes or until noodles are soft. Strain noodles and top with basil, almonds, parsley and garlic. Toss with olive oil and sprinkle salt to taste. | | |
| | Drink | Water |
| Snack 2 | | Protein bar, no more than 220 calories and 5 g of fat |
| | Drink | Water |
| Meal 3 – lemon and ginger salmon | | |
| 6 oz. salmon | | Lemon and fresh ginger |
| Top salmon with lemon and fresh ginger and fold tightly in tinfoil. Bake at 350 for approximately 20 -25 min | | |
| | Side | 1 cup steamed vegetables |
| | Drinks | Water |

# Fit Shred

# Keep pushing your almost there, stay focused! Drink plenty of water!!!

## Week 5 Day3

| Meal 1 – Blueberry oat pancakes 1 serving is 3 pancakes | |
|---|---|
| 1 cup old fashioned oats | 2 large eggs |
| 1 cup blue berries | 1 tsp. vanilla extract |
| ½ cup low fat cottage cheese | 1 tsp. 100% maple syrup or 2/3 cup light Greek yogurt |
| In a blender, combine oats, cottage cheese, eggs and vanilla extract. Stir in blueberries. Scoop batter onto warm skillet and make 3-inch pancakes. Cook until brown on each side. Top with maple syrup or Greek yogurt. | |

| | Drink | Water |
|---|---|---|
| Snack 1 | | 1 cup apple sliced-1 ½ tbsp. natural peanut butter |
| | Drink | Water |

| Meal 2 – chicken wrap | |
|---|---|
| 6-inch whole grain tortilla | Red bell pepper, sliced |
| 3oz. grilled chicken breast | Lettuce |
| Tomato, sliced | |
| preheat oven to 450. Top pizza crust with all ingredients and bake until crispy, approximately 6-10 minutes. | |

| | Side | Celery sticks 1 tbsp. low fat ranch dressing |
|---|---|---|
| | Drink | Water |
| Snack 2 | | 1 cup low fat cottage cheese- 1 servings of fruit |
| | Drink | Water |

| Meal 3 – marinated turkey | |
|---|---|
| 4oz marinated turkey tenderloin | ½ cup long grain and wild rice |
| Marinate turkey tenderloin in your favorite sauce for 20 minutes. Bake at 350 for 30 minutes or cook over medium heat for approximately 10 minutes on each side. | |

| | Side | 1 cup green peas 1 cup fresh fruit. |
|---|---|---|
| | Drinks | Water |

## Week 5 day 4

| Meal 1 – shake | | |
|---|---|---|
| 1 scoop whey protein | | ½ cup water |
| 1 whole banana | | Handful of ice |
| ½ cup skim, almond, or rice milk | | |
| | Drink | Water |
| Snack 1 | | ½ cup almonds, cashews, dried cranberries |
| | Drink | Water |

| Meal 2 – spinach and quinoa salad | | |
|---|---|---|
| 1 lb. of baby spinach | | 1/3 cup olive oil |
| 1 ½ cups quinoa | | 8oz crumble feta |
| ½ cup red wine vinegar | | Salt and pepper |
| Cook quinoa in 3 cups of boiling water. Cover and simmer for 15-20 minutes. Combine all liquids ingredients then add spinach and warm quinoa. Top with feta an enjoy. | | |
| | Side | 1 medium size fruit |
| | Drink | Water |
| Snack 2 | | Smoothie ¾ cup plain, fat free yogurt<br>½ cup frozen mixed berries<br>1 medium banana<br>¼ cup skim milk |
| | Drink | Water |

| Meal 3 – south western pizza1 serving is 2 slices | | |
|---|---|---|
| 12" whole wheat pizza crust | | 1 ¼ cups reduced fat mozzarella cheese, shredded |
| 2 scallions, thinly sliced | | 1/4cup cilantro leaves |
| 1 1/3 cups canned black beans | | 1 small red pepper, chopped |
| 1 cup tomatoes | | |
| Top pizza crust with all ingredients. Bake at 450 for 8-10 minutes | | |
| | Drinks | Water |

## Week 5 Day 5

| Meal 1 – Oatmeal | | |
|---|---|---|
| 2/3 cup oatmeal (non-instant) | | 2tsp. maple syrup or natural sweetener |
| | Side | ½ cup of milk or yogurt |
| | Drink | Water |
| Snack 1 | | 6 0z. light Greek yogurt |
| | Drink | Water |
| Meal 2 – soup and salad | | |
| 1 ½ cups broth-based soup | | 2 cups tossed greens with vegetables |
| ¼ cup cottage cheese or non-fat dressing | | |
| | Drink | Water |
| Snack 2 | | Protein bar, no more than 220 calories and 5g of fat. |
| | Drink | Water |
| Meal 3 – Lemon and Ginger Salmon | | |
| 6 oz salmon | | Lemon and fresh ginger |
| Top salmon with lemon and fresh ginger and fold tightly in tinfoil. Bake at 350 for about 20-25 minutes. | | |
| | Side | 1 cup steamed vegetables 1cup quinoa |
| | Drink | Water |

## Week 5 Day 6

| Meal 1 – Cereal | | |
|---|---|---|
| 1 cup non-sweetened whole grain cereal 1 cup water | | 1 cup of low fat milk |
| | Side | 1 serving of fruit |
| | Drink | Water |
| Snack 1 | | 10 – 15 baby carrots -2 tbsp low fat ranch dressing |
| | Drink | Water |

| Meal 2 – whole wheat sandwich | | |
| --- | --- | --- |
| 2 slices whole wheat or Ezekiel bread | | 1 tbsp. light miracle whip or light mayo/mustard |
| 4 slices lean turkey or another lean deli meat | | Tomato, lettuce, or others to taste |
| | Drink | Water |
| Snack 2 | | 1 banana, 1 handful of nuts |
| | Drink | Water |
| Meal 3 – feta chicken salad | | |
| 6 oz cooked chicken breast, sliced | | Feta cheese, shredded lettuce |
| Shredded lettuce with cooked chicken. Sprinkled with feta cheese | | |
| | Side | 1 serving of fruit |
| | Drink | Water |

## Week 5 Day 7

| Meal 1 – shake and oatmeal | | |
| --- | --- | --- |
| 1 scoop of whey protein | | ½ cup skim, almond, or rice milk |
| 1 whole banana | | Ice |
| ½ cup of water | | 2/3 cup oatmeal 2tsp maple syrup |
| | Side | ½ cup of milk or yogurt |
| | Drink | Water |
| Snack 1 | | ½ cup low-fat cottage cheese – 1 cup fruit |
| | Drink | Water |
| Meal 2 – turkey pita | | |
| 1 large wheat pita | | 1 tbsp. light miracle whip or light mayonnaise |
| 4 slices lean turkey or another lean deli meat | | ½ tbsp. mustard |
| 1 oz. slice of cheese | | Tomato, cucumber, lettuce, sprouts, other vegetables |
| Spread miracle whip and mustard on the pita. Fill pita with meat, cheese and vegetables. | | |
| | Side | 4 celery sticks, 1 cup raw broccoli, 2 tbsp. low-fat dressing |
| | Drink | Water |

| Snack 2 | | 1 serving of fruit<br>1 part-skim mozzarella string cheese |
|---|---|---|
| | Drink | Water |

| Meal 3 – grilled teriyaki tuna | |
|---|---|
| 4 oz. tuna steak | 1/3 cup cooked brown rice |
| 2 tbsp. low-fat, bottled teriyaki sauce | Fresh spinach 1 tsp. olive oil |
| Place tuna steak in saucepan with olive oil. Cook approximately 10 minutes or until meat is done. Add teriyaki sauce and place on top of rice with a side of fresh spinach. | |

| | Drink | Water |
|---|---|---|

## Week 6 day 1

| Meal 1 – Blueberry Oat Pancakes | |
|---|---|
| 1 cup old fashioned oats | 2 large eggs |
| 1 cup blueberries | 1 tsp. vanilla extract |
| ½ cup low-fat cottage cheese | 1 tsp. 100% maple syrup or 2/3 cup of light reek yogurt. |
| In a blender, combine oats, cottage cheese, eggs and vanilla extract. Stir in blueberries. Scoop batter onto warm skillet and make 3-4-inch pancakes. Cook until brown on each side. Top with maple syrup or Greek yogurt. | |

| | Drink | Water |
|---|---|---|
| Snack 1 | | 1 serving of fruit -1 string cheese |
| | Drink | Water |

| Meal 2 – grilled chicken | |
|---|---|
| 6oz chicken breast | 2 cups tossed greens with vegetables |
| Top chicken breast with your favorite herbs and spices. Bake at 350 for 20-30 minutes or grill tor approximately 20 minutes. | |
| 4 cups tossed greens with vegetables ½ cup cottage cheese | |

| | Drink | Water |
|---|---|---|
| Snack 2 | | ¼ cup cottage cheese- 1 serving of fruit |
| | Drink | Water |

| Meal 3 – stir fry | |
|---|---|
| 1 cup cooked rice | 1 ½ cups vegetables |

| 1 cup light coconut milk | Curry spice to taste |
| --- | --- |
| Place vegetables in saucepan. Add milk and curry spice. Cook until vegetables are done then place mixture on top of cooked rice. | |
| | Drink | Water |

## Week 6 day 2

| Meal 1 – Blueberry Oat Pancakes | |
| --- | --- |
| 1 cup old fashioned oats | 2 large eggs |
| 1 cup blueberries | 1 tsp. vanilla extract |
| ½ cup low-fat cottage cheese | 1 tsp. 100% maple syrup or 2/3 cup of light reek yogurt. |
| In a blender, combine oats, cottage cheese, eggs and vanilla extract. Stir in blueberries. Scoop batter onto warm skillet and make 3-4-inch pancakes. Cook until brown on each side. Top with maple syrup or Greek yogurt. | |
| | Drink | Water |
| Snack 1 | 1 serving of fruit -1 string cheese |
| Drink | Drink | Water |

| Meal 2 – grilled chicken | |
| --- | --- |
| 6oz chicken breast | 2 cups tossed greens with vegetables |
| Top chicken breast with your favorite herbs and spices. Bake at 350 for 20-30 minutes or grill tor approximately 20 minutes. | |
| 4 cups tossed greens with vegetables ½ cup cottage cheese | |
| | Drink | Water |
| Snack 2 | ¼ cup cottage cheese- 1 serving of fruit |
| | Drink | Water |

| Meal 3 – stir fry | |
| --- | --- |
| 1 cup cooked rice | 1 ½ cups vegetables |
| 1 cup light coconut milk | Curry spice to taste |
| Place vegetables in saucepan. Add milk and curry spice. Cook until vegetables are done then place mixture on top of cooked rice. | |
| | Drink | Water |

## Week 6 Day 3

| Meal 1 – Oatmeal | | |
|---|---|---|
| 2/3 cup oatmeal (non-instant) | | 2tsp. maple syrup or natural sweetener |
| | Side | ½ cup of milk or yogurt |
| | Drink | Water |
| Snack 1 | | 6 0z. light Greek yogurt |
| | Drink | Water |
| Meal 2 – soup and salad | | |
| 1 ½ cups broth-based soup | | 2 cups tossed greens with vegetables |
| ¼ cup cottage cheese or non-fat dressing | | |
| | Drink | Water |
| Snack 2 | | Protein bar, no more than 220 calories and 5g of fat. |
| | Drink | Water |
| Meal 3 – Lemon and Ginger Salmon | | |
| 6 oz salmon | | Lemon and fresh ginger |
| Top salmon with lemon and fresh ginger and fold tightly in tinfoil. Bake at 350 for about 20-25 minutes. | | |
| | Side | 1 cup steamed vegetables 1cup quinoa |
| | Drink | Water |

## Week 6 Day 4

| Meal 1 – Cereal | | |
|---|---|---|
| 1 cup non-sweetened whole grain cereal<br>1 cup water | | 1 cup of low fat milk |
| | Side | 1 serving of fruit |
| | Drink | Water |
| Snack 1 | | 10 – 15 baby carrots -2 tbsp low fat ranch dressing |
| | Drink | Water |
| Meal 2 – whole wheat sandwich | | |

| | | |
|---|---|---|
| 2 slices whole wheat or Ezekiel bread | | 1 tbsp. light miracle whip or light mayo/mustard |
| 4 slices lean turkey or another lean deli meat | | Tomato, lettuce, or others to taste |
| | Drink | Water |
| Snack 2 | | 1 banana, 1 handful of nuts |
| | Drink | Water |
| **Meal 3 – feta chicken salad** | | |
| 6 oz cooked chicken breast, sliced | | Feta cheese, shredded lettuce |
| Shredded lettuce with cooked chicken. Sprinkled with feta cheese | | |
| | Side | 1 serving of fruit |
| | Drink | Water |

## Week 6 Day 5

| | | |
|---|---|---|
| **Meal 1 – Blueberry Oat Pancakes** | | |
| 1 cup old fashioned oats | | 2 large eggs |
| 1 cup blueberries | | 1 tsp. vanilla extract |
| ½ cup low-fat cottage cheese | | 1 tsp. 100% maple syrup or 2/3 cup of light reek yogurt. |
| In a blender, combine oats, cottage cheese, eggs and vanilla extract. Stir in blueberries. Scoop batter onto warm skillet and make 3-4-inch pancakes. Cook until brown on each side. Top with maple syrup or Greek yogurt. | | |
| | Drink | Water |
| Snack 1 | | 1 serving of fruit -1 string cheese |
| | Drink | Water |
| **Meal 2 – grilled chicken** | | |
| 6oz chicken breast | | 2 cups tossed greens with vegetables |
| Top chicken breast with your favorite herbs and spices. Bake at 350 for 20-30 minutes or grill tor approximately 20 minutes. | | |
| 4 cups tossed greens with vegetables ½ cup cottage cheese | | |
| | Drink | Water |
| Snack 2 | | ¼ cup cottage cheese- 1 serving of fruit |
| | Drink | Water |
| **Meal 3 – stir fry** | | |

| | |
|---|---|
| 1 cup cooked rice | 1 ½ cups vegetables |
| 1 cup light coconut milk | Curry spice to taste |
| Place vegetables in saucepan. Add milk and curry spice. Cook until vegetables are done then place mixture on top of cooked rice. | |

| | Drink | Water |
|---|---|---|

## Week 6 Day 6

| Meal 1 – veggie egg white omelet | | |
|---|---|---|
| 4 – 5 egg whites | | 1 plum tomato, chopped |
| 1 egg yolk | | 1 small clove of garlic, chopped |
| 2 tbsp. skim milk | | 1 handful spinach, shredded |
| 1 tbsp. onion, minced | | Lite cooking spray |
| Place eggs, milk, vegetables add garlic in bowl or blender and mix together. Spray large skillet with cooking spray and place mixture in pan. Cook on both sides until done. | | |
| | Drink | Water |
| Snack 1 | | 1 cup grapes – ¼ cup almonds |
| | Drink | Water |
| Meal 2 – Avocado and chicken salad | | |
| 4 oz. grilled chicken | | ½ cup orange, sliced |
| 3 cup mixed greens | | 1 tbsp. lemon juice |
| ¼ cup avocado, sliced | | 2 tsp. olive oil |
| Top mixed greens with orange, avocado and chicken. Drizzle with olive oil and lemon juice. | | |
| | Drink | Water |
| Snack 2 | | 10 – 15 baby carrots- 2tbsp. low-fat ranch dip |
| | Drink | Water |
| Meal 3 – BLT with Turkey | | |
| 2 slices whole wheat bread | | Tomato, sliced |
| 3 slices turkey bacon | | Lettuce, to taste |
| | Sides | 1 serving of fruit |
| | Drink | water |

## Week 6 Day 7

| Meal 1 – Blueberry Oat Pancakes | | |
|---|---|---|
| 1 cup old fashioned oats | | 2 large eggs |
| 1 cup blueberries | | 1 tsp. vanilla extract |
| ½ cup low-fat cottage cheese | | 1 tsp. 100% maple syrup or 2/3 cup of light reek yogurt. |
| In a blender, combine oats, cottage cheese, eggs and vanilla extract. Stir in blueberries. Scoop batter onto warm skillet and make 3-4-inch pancakes. Cook until brown on each side. Top with maple syrup or Greek yogurt. | | |
| | Drink | Water |
| Snack 1 | | 1 serving of fruit -1 string cheese |
| | Drink | Water |
| Meal 2 – minestrone soup | | |
| 1 ½ cups low sodium minestrone soup | | 1 whole grain roll or toast |
| | Side | 1 tomato, sliced 1 oz. mozzarella, sliced basil and balsamic vinegar |
| | Drink | Water |
| Snack 2 | | 1 cup grapes – ¼ cup almonds |
| | Drink | Water |
| Meal 3 – Roast beef pita | | |
| 4 oz. lean roast beef or other lean meat | | Dark salad greens |
| 3 – inch whole wheat pita | | Bell peppers, sliced |
| Cherry tomatoes, sliced | | Cucumbers, sliced |
| Romaine lettuce | | Mushrooms, sliced |
| | Drink | Water |

## Week 7 Day 1

| Meal 1 – egg burrito | |
|---|---|
| 4 small whole grain tortillas | ½ cup sweet onion, chopped |
| 2 cups egg white | Salt and pepper |
| ½ cup low-fat cottage cheese | ½ cup black beans |
| ½ cup tomatoes, chopped | Lite cooking spray |

| | | |
|---|---|---|
| ½ cup red or green sweet pepper, chopped | | |
| Spray large skillet with cooking spray. Add eggs, cottage cheese, vegetables and beans. Stir together. Once fully cooked, place mixture on tortillas. Salt and pepper to taste. | | |
| | Side | ½ cup milk or yogurt |
| | Drink | Water |
| Snack 1 | | 2 slices turkey jerky |
| | Drink | Water |
| **Meal 2 – Meatballs and Marinara** | | |
| 4oz. extra-lean ground turkey | | 2 tbsp. parmesan cheese, grated |
| ½ cup marinara sauce | | Lite cooking spray |
| Roll ground turkey into 3-4 balls. Spray pan with cooking spray and cook meatballs approximately 7 minutes. Top meatballs with marinara sauce and parmesan cheese. | | |
| | Drink | Water |
| Snack 2 | | 6 oz. light Greek yogurt |
| | Drink | Water |
| **Meal 3 – bagel sandwich** | | |
| ½ whole wheat bagel or 1 slice toast | | 1 slice reduced fat cheese |
| 2 oz. deli style turkey breast, sliced | | Tomato, sliced |
| | Drink | Water |

## Week 7 day 2

| | | |
|---|---|---|
| **Meal 1 – oatmeal** | | |
| 2/3 cup old fashioned oats | | 2 tsp. 100% maple syrup or natural sweetener |
| 1 cup water | | |
| Follow oatmeal instructions and top with maple syrup. | | |
| | Side | ½ cup milk or yogurt |
| | Drink | Water |
| Snack 1 | | 6oz light Greek yogurt or kefir |
| | Drink | Water |
| **Meal 2 – peanut butter and banana** | | |
| 1 slice whole grain or Ezekiel bread | | 1 tbsp. all fruit preserves or banana |

| | | |
|---|---|---|
| 1 tbsp. natural peanut butter | | |
| | Drink | Water |
| Snack 2 | | Protein bar, no more than 220 calories and 5 g of fat |
| | Drink | Water |
| **Meal 3 – turkey burger** | | |
| 4oz. lean ground turkey | | 2 tbsp. red onion, chopped |
| 2 tbsp. salsa | | 1 whole grain pita |
| Form ground turkey into a patty. Cook turkey approximately 4 minutes on each side until done. Top with salsa and onion and place in whole grain pita. | | |
| | Side | 1 cup steamed vegetables |
| | Drinks | Water |

## Week 7 day 3

| | | |
|---|---|---|
| **Meal 1 – oatmeal** | | |
| 2/3 cup old fashioned oats | | 2 tsp. 100% maple syrup or natural sweetener |
| 1 cup water | | |
| Follow oatmeal instructions and top with maple syrup. | | |
| | Side | ½ cup milk or yogurt |
| | Drink | Water |
| Snack 1 | | 6oz light Greek yogurt or kefir |
| | Drink | Water |
| **Meal 2 – peanut butter and banana** | | |
| 1 slice whole grain or Ezekiel bread | | 1 tbsp. all fruit preserves or banana |
| 1 tbsp. natural peanut butter | | |
| | Drink | Water |
| Snack 2 | | Protein bar, no more than 220 calories and 5 g of fat |
| | Drink | Water |
| **Meal 3 – turkey burger** | | |
| 4oz. lean ground turkey | | 2 tbsp. red onion, chopped |
| 2 tbsp. salsa | | 1 whole grain pita |
| Form ground turkey into a patty. Cook turkey approximately 4 minutes on each side until done. Top with salsa and onion and place in whole grain pita. | | |

| | Side | 1 cup steamed vegetables |
| --- | --- | --- |
| | Drinks | Water |

## Week 7 day 4

| Meal 1 – cereal | | |
| --- | --- | --- |
| 1 cup non-sweetened whole grain cereal | | 1 cup low-fat milk |
| | Drink | Water |
| Snack 1 | | ½ cup low-fat cottage cheese- 1 serving of fruit. |
| | Drink | Water |
| Meal 2 – grilled chicken salad | | |
| 3oz grilled chicken breast | | 1 tbsp. pecans, chopped |
| 3 cups mixed dark greens | | Cucumber, sliced |
| ½ apple, chopped | | |
| Top mixed greens with chicken, chopped apple, pecans and cucumber to taste. | | |
| | Drink | Water |
| Snack 2 | | 1 banana- 1 handful nuts |
| | Drink | Water |
| Meal 3 – marinated turkey | | |
| 4oz. marinated turkey tenderloins | | ½ cup long grain and wild rice |
| Marinate turkey tenderloin in your favorite sauce for 20 minutes. Bake at 350 for 30 minutes or cook over medium heat for approximately 10 minutes on each side or until done. | | |
| | Side | ½ cup green peas 1 cup fresh fruit. |
| | Drink | Water |

## Week 7 day 5

| Meal 1 – buckwheat cereal | | |
| --- | --- | --- |
| 2/3 cup buckwheat cereal | | ½ banana |
| 1 cup water | | 1 tsp. 100% maple syrup |
| Mix buckwheat cereal with water and cook for 20 minutes on the stove, top with banana and syrup. | | |
| | Drink | 1 cup of milk |

# Pioneerfit Athletica

| Snack 1 | | 1 serving of fruit -1 mozzarella string cheese |
|---|---|---|
| | Drink | Water |
| **Meal 2 – grilled chicken wrap** | | |
| 6-inch whole grain tortilla | | Red bell pepper, sliced |
| 3 oz. grilled chicken breast | | Lettuce |
| Tomato, sliced | | |
| | Side | Celery sticks 1 tbsp. low fat ranch dressing |
| | Drink | Water |
| Snack 2 | | ¼ cup cottage cheese- 1 serving of fruit |
| | Drink | Water |
| **Meal 3 – lemon chicken** | | |
| 6 oz. chicken breast | | 1 ½ cups vegetables |
| 1 lemon | | |
| Squeeze lemon juice over chicken. Bake at 350 for 20-30 minutes. Bake assorted vegetables at 350 for 10-15 minutes. | | |
| | Side | ½ cup fresh fruit |
| | Drink | Water |

## Week 7 day 6

| **Meal 1 – shake** | | |
|---|---|---|
| 1 scoop whey protein | | 1 tsp. peanut butter |
| ½ cup fat free milk | | Handful of ice |
| ½ cup water | | |
| | Drink | Water |
| Snack 1 | | 10 -15 baby carrots- 2tbsp. low fat ranch dip |
| | Drink | Water |
| **Meal 2 – turkey pita** | | |
| 1 large wheat pita | | 1 tbsp. light miracle whip or light mayo |
| 4 slices lean turkey | | Tomato, cucumber, lettuce, sprouts or another veg. |
| 1 oz. slice of cheese | | ½ tbsp. mustard |

| | | |
|---|---|---|
| Spread miracle whip and mustard on the pita. Fill pita with turkey, cheese and vegetables. | | |
| | Side | 4 celery sticks 1 cup raw broccoli 2 tbsp. low fat dressing |
| | Drink | Water |
| Snack 2 | | 1 serving of fruit – 1-part skim mozzarella string cheese |
| | Drink | Water |
| **Meal 3 – meaty turkey burger 1 burger per serving** | | |
| 1 lb. extra lean ground turkey | | ¼ cup low fat chicken or vegetable stock |
| ½ cup oat bran | | 1 clove of garlic, pressed |
| 2 tbsp. flaxseed | | 1 tbsp. soy sauce |
| 2 egg whites | | 1 whole wheat bun |
| Mix ground turkey with oat bran, flaxseed, egg whites, stock, garlic and soy sauce. Form into 3 patties and cook approximately 5 minutes on each side or until done. Place on whole wheat bun. | | |
| | Side | 1 cup steamed vegetables |
| | Drink | Water |

## Week 7 day 7

| | | |
|---|---|---|
| **Meal 1 – veggie egg white omelet** | | |
| 4-5 egg whites | | 1 plum tomato, chopped |
| 1 egg yolk | | 1 small clove of garlic, chopped |
| 2 tbsp. skim milk | | 1 handful spinach, shredded |
| 1 tbsp. onion, minced | | Lite cooking spray |
| Place eggs, milk, vegetables and garlic in bowl or blender and mix together. Spray large skillet with cooking spray and place mixture in pan. Cook on both sides until done. | | |
| | Drink | Water |
| Snack 1 | | 1 cup grapes- ¼ cup almonds |
| | Drink | Water |
| **Meal 2 – avocado and chicken salad** | | |
| 4 oz. grilled chicken | | ½ cup orange, sliced |
| 3 cups mixed greens | | 1 tbsp. lemon juice |
| ¼ cup avocado, sliced | | 2 tsp. olive oil |

| | | |
|---|---|---|
| Top mixed greens with orange, avocado and chicken. Drizzle with olive oil and lemon juice. breast with your favorite herbs and spices. | | |
| | Drink | Water |
| Snack 2 | | ¼ cup cottage cheese- 1 serving of fruit |
| | Drink | Water |
| **Meal 3 – black bean soup and sandwich** | | |
| 1 cup of canned black bean soup | | 2 thin sliced avocados |
| 1 slice whole grain bread | | 1 tsp. Dijon mustard |
| 2 oz. deli style turkey breast, sliced | | |
| Spread Dijon mustard over bread. Top with turkey and avocado | | |
| | Drink | Water |

## Week 8 day 1

| | | |
|---|---|---|
| **Meal 1 – Blueberry Oat Pancakes** | | |
| 1 cup old fashioned oats | | 2 large eggs |
| 1 cup blueberries | | 1 tsp. vanilla extract |
| ½ cup low-fat cottage cheese | | 1 tsp. 100% maple syrup or 2/3 cup of light reek yogurt. |
| In a blender, combine oats, cottage cheese, eggs and vanilla extract. Stir in blueberries. Scoop batter onto warm skillet and make 3-4-inch pancakes. Cook until brown on each side. Top with maple syrup or Greek yogurt. | | |
| | Drink | Water |
| Snack 1 | | 1 serving of fruit -1 string cheese |
| | Drink | Water |
| **Meal 2 – grilled chicken** | | |
| 6oz chicken breast | | 2 cups tossed greens with vegetables |
| Top chicken breast with your favorite herbs and spices. Bake at 350 for 20-30 minutes or grill tor approximately 20 minutes. | | |
| 4 cups tossed greens with vegetables ½ cup cottage cheese | | |
| | Drink | Water |
| Snack 2 | | ¼ cup cottage cheese- 1 serving of fruit |
| | Drink | Water |
| **Meal 3 – stir fry** | | |
| 1 cup cooked rice | | 1 ½ cups vegetables |

| | |
|---|---|
| 1 cup light coconut milk | Curry spice to taste |
| Place vegetables in saucepan. Add milk and curry spice. Cook until vegetables are done then place mixture on top of cooked rice. ||

| | Drink | Water |
|---|---|---|

## Week 8 day 2

| Meal 1 – egg burrito ||
|---|---|
| 4 small whole grain tortillas | ½ cup sweet onion, chopped |
| 2 cups egg whites | ½ cup black beans |
| ½ cup low-fat cottage cheese | Salt and pepper |
| ½ cup tomatoes, chopped | Lite cooking spray |
| ½ cup red or green sweet pepper, chopped. | |
| Spray large skillet with cooking spray. Add eggs, cottage cheese, vegetables and beans. Stir together. Once fully cooked, place mixture on tortillas. Salt and pepper to taste. ||

| | Drink | Water |
|---|---|---|
| Snack 1 | | 2 slices of turkey jerky |
| | Drink | Water |

| Meal 2 – meatballs and marinara ||
|---|---|
| 4 oz. extra lean | 2 tbsp. parmesan cheese, grated |
| ½ cup marinara sauce | Lite cooking spray |
| Roll ground turkey into 3 -4 balls. Spray pan with cooking spray and cook meatballs approximately 7 minutes. Top meatballs with marinara sauce and parmesan cheese. ||

| | Drink | Water |
|---|---|---|
| Snack 2 | | 6 oz. light Greek yogurt |
| | Drink | Water |

| Meal 3 – rosemary chicken ||
|---|---|
| 4 oz chicken | 2 cups arugula |
| 1tsp. rosemary | 1tbsp. parmesan cheese grated |
| ½ tsp. garlic, minced | 1 tsp. olive oil |
| Top chicken with rosemary, garlic and olive oil. Wrap in tin foil and bake at 350 for 20 minutes or until fully cooked. Top arugula with the chicken and sprinkle with parmesan cheese. ||

| | | |
|---|---|---|
| | Side | 1 cup of beets |
| | Drink | Water |

## Week 8 day 3

| Meal 1 – egg burrito | |
|---|---|
| 4 small whole grain tortillas | ½ cup sweet onion, chopped |
| 2 cups egg whites | ½ cup black beans |
| ½ cup low-fat cottage cheese | Salt and pepper |
| ½ cup tomatoes, chopped | Lite cooking spray |
| ½ cup red or green sweet pepper, chopped. | |
| Spray large skillet with cooking spray. Add eggs, cottage cheese, vegetables and beans. Stir together. Once fully cooked, place mixture on tortillas. Salt and pepper to taste. | |

| | | |
|---|---|---|
| | Drink | Water |
| Snack 1 | | 2 slices of turkey jerky |
| | Drink | Water |

| Meal 2 – meatballs and marinara | |
|---|---|
| 4 oz. extra lean | 2 tbsp. parmesan cheese, grated |
| ½ cup marinara sauce | Lite cooking spray |
| Roll ground turkey into 3 -4 balls. Spray pan with cooking spray and cook meatballs approximately 7 minutes. Top meatballs with marinara sauce and parmesan cheese. | |

| | | |
|---|---|---|
| | Drink | Water |
| Snack 2 | | 6 oz. light Greek yogurt |
| | Drink | Water |

| Meal 3 – rosemary chicken | |
|---|---|
| 4 oz chicken | 2 cups arugula |
| 1tsp. rosemary | 1tbsp. parmesan cheese grated |
| ½ tsp. garlic, minced | 1 tsp. olive oil |
| Top chicken with rosemary, garlic and olive oil. Wrap in tin foil and bake at 350 for 20 minutes or until fully cooked. Top arugula with the chicken and sprinkle with parmesan cheese. | |

| | | |
|---|---|---|
| | Side | 1 cup of beets |
| | Drink | Water |

## Week 8 day 4

| Meal 1 – oatmeal | | |
|---|---|---|
| 2/3 cup old fashioned oats | | 2 tsp. 100% maple syrup or natural sweetener |
| 1 cup water | | |
| Follow oatmeal instructions and top with maple syrup. | | |
| | Side | ½ cup milk or yogurt |
| | Drink | Water |
| Snack 1 | | 6oz light Greek yogurt or kefir |
| | Drink | Water |
| Meal 2 – peanut butter and banana | | |
| 1 slice whole grain or Ezekiel bread | | 1 tbsp. all fruit preserves or banana |
| 1 tbsp. natural peanut butter | | |
| | Drink | Water |
| Snack 2 | | Protein bar, no more than 220 calories and 5 g of fat |
| | Drink | Water |
| Meal 3 – turkey burger | | |
| 4oz. lean ground turkey | | 2 tbsp. red onion, chopped |
| 2 tbsp. salsa | | 1 whole grain pita |
| Form ground turkey into a patty. Cook turkey approximately 4 minutes on each side until done. Top with salsa and onion and place in whole grain pita. | | |
| | Side | 1 cup steamed vegetables |
| | Drinks | Water |

## Week 8 Day 5

| Meal 1 – turkey bacon on toast | | |
|---|---|---|
| 3 slices of turkey bacon | | 1 slice Ezekiel bread, toasted |
| ½ tomato, sliced | | |
| | Drink | Water |
| Snack 1 | | 10 raw almonds |
| | Drink | Water |
| Pesto spaghetti 1 ½ cup per serving | | |
| 1lb. buckwheat or rice noodles | | ½ cup almonds, chopped |

| 3 quarts water | ¾ cup parsley |
| --- | --- |
| 1 tsp. salt | 2 cloves of garlic, chopped |
| 3 cups fresh basil leaves | Extra virgin olive oil |
| Boil noodles in water and salt approximately 12 minutes or until noodles are soft. Strain noodles and top with basil, almonds, parsley and garlic. Toss with olive oil and sprinkle salt to taste. | |
| | Drink | Water |

| Snack 2 | | Protein bar, no more than 220 calories and 5 g of fat |
| --- | --- | --- |
| | Drink | Water |

| Meal 3 – lemon and ginger salmon | |
| --- | --- |
| 6 oz. salmon | Lemon and fresh ginger |
| Top salmon with lemon and fresh ginger and fold tightly in tinfoil. Bake at 350 for approximately 20 -25 min | |
| | Side | 1 cup steamed vegetables |
| | Drinks | Water |

## Week 8 day 6

## Week 8 Day 7

| Meal 1 – Blueberry oat pancakes 1 serving is 3 pancakes | |
| --- | --- |
| 1 cup old fashioned oats | 2 large eggs |
| 1 cup blue berries | 1 tsp. vanilla extract |
| ½ cup low fat cottage cheese | 1 tsp. 100% maple syrup or 2/3 cup light Greek yogurt |
| In a blender, combine oats, cottage cheese, eggs and vanilla extract. Stir in blueberries. Scoop batter onto warm skillet and make 3-inch pancakes. Cook until brown on each side. Top with maple syrup or Greek yogurt. | |
| | Drink | Water |

| Snack 1 | | 1 cup apple sliced-1 ½ tbsp. natural peanut butter |
| --- | --- | --- |
| | Drink | Water |

| Meal 2 – chicken wrap | |
| --- | --- |
| 6-inch whole grain tortilla | Red bell pepper, sliced |
| 3oz. grilled chicken breast | Lettuce |

| | | |
|---|---|---|
| Tomato, sliced | | |
| preheat oven to 450. Top pizza crust with all ingredients and bake until crispy, approximately 6-10 minutes. | | |
| | Side | Celery sticks 1 tbsp. low fat ranch dressing |
| | Drink | Water |
| Snack 2 | | 1 cup low fat cottage cheese- 1 servings of fruit |
| | Drink | Water |
| **Meal 3 – marinated turkey** | | |
| 4oz marinated turkey tenderloin | | ½ cup long grain and wild rice |
| Marinate turkey tenderloin in your favorite sauce for 20 minutes. Bake at 350 for 30 minutes or cook over medium heat for approximately 10 minutes on each side. | | |
| | Side | 1 cup green peas 1 cup fresh fruit. |
| | Drinks | Water |
| **Meal 1 – shake** | | |
| 1 scoop whey protein | | ½ cup water |
| 1 whole banana | | Handful of ice |
| ½ cup skim, almond, or rice milk | | |
| | Drink | Water |
| Snack 1 | | ½ cup almonds, cashews, dried cranberries |
| | Drink | Water |
| **Meal 2 – spinach and quinoa salad** | | |
| 1 lb. of baby spinach | | 1/3 cup olive oil |
| 1 ½ cups quinoa | | 8oz crumble feta |
| ½ cup red wine vinegar | | Salt and pepper |
| Cook quinoa in 3 cups of boiling water. Cover and simmer for 15-20 minutes. Combine all liquids ingredients then add spinach and warm quinoa. Top with feta an enjoy. | | |
| | Side | 1 medium size fruit |
| | Drink | Water |

| | | |
|---|---|---|
| Snack 2 | | Smoothie ¾ cup plain, fat free yogurt<br>½ cup frozen mixed berries<br>1 medium banana<br>¼ cup skim milk |
| | Drink | Water |
| **Meal 3 – south western pizza1 serving is 2 slices** | | |
| 12" whole wheat pizza crust | | 1 ¼ cups reduced fat mozzarella cheese, shredded |
| 2 scallions, thinly sliced | | 1/4cup cilantro leaves |
| 1 1/3 cups canned black beans | | 1 small red pepper, chopped |
| 1 cup tomatoes | | |
| Top pizza crust with all ingredients. Bake at 450 for 8-10 minutes | | |
| | Drinks | Water |

Monday Functional High
Intensity Training workout

Week 1 pre-training

**2 x 7** min
circuits

**14** min
workout time

**37** min
total time

## Warm up -10 min

## F.H.I.T Circuit - 7 min - Repeat 2 times

### 1 Sumo Squats x30

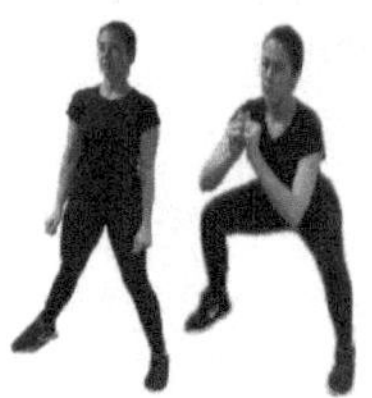

### 2 high Knees 1min

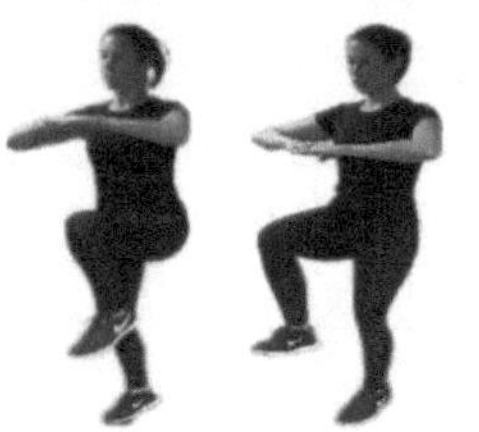

### 3 leg scissors x25

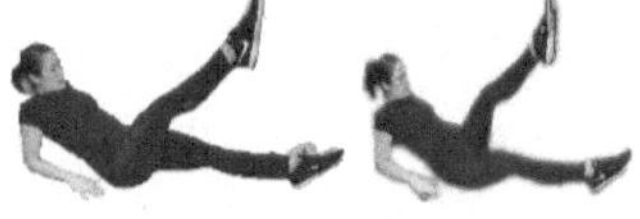

### 4 butt kicks

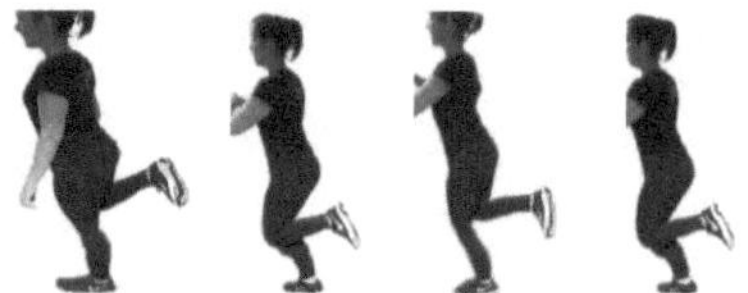

### 5 Triceps dips x25

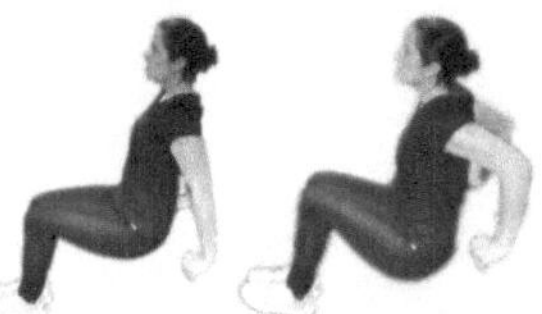

### 6 Abdominal bicycle x30

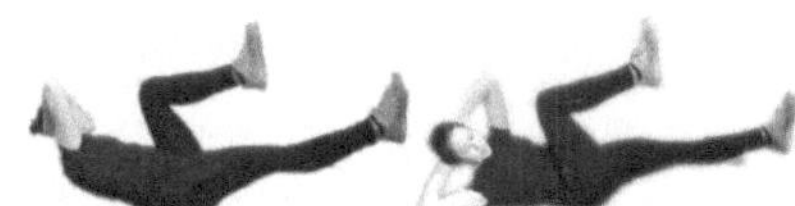

### 7 Side shuffles 1 min

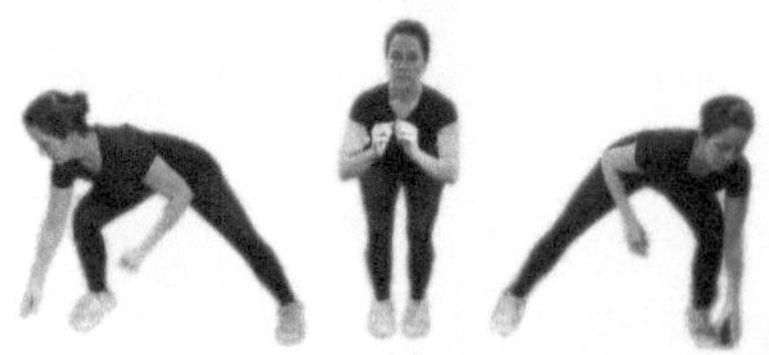

Rest period between circuit rounds 2 min then begin circuits again.

Cool down – 10 min- see page

Tuesday is recovery training

Week 1 pre-training

**2 x 5** min
warmup & cool down

**30** min
workout time

**40** min
total time

## Warm up -5 min

## Cardio - 30 min

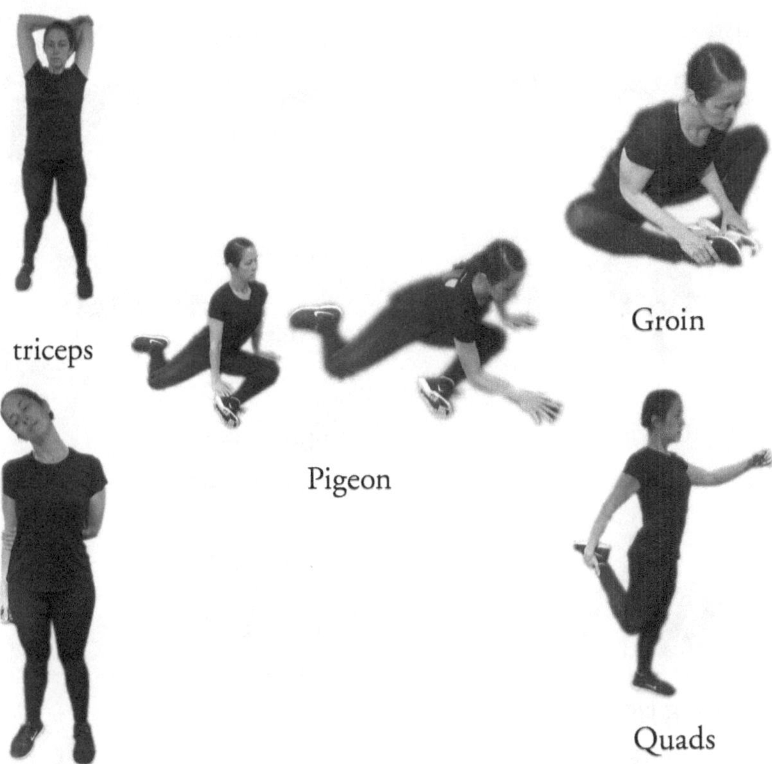


Make sure to follow stretches on page

Cool down – 5 min- see page

Wednesday Functional High Intensity Training workout
Week 1 pre-training

**2 x 7** min
circuits

**14** min
workout time

**37** min
total time

## Warm up -10 min

## F.H.I.T Circuit - 7 min - Repeat 2 times

### 1 Push Ups x20

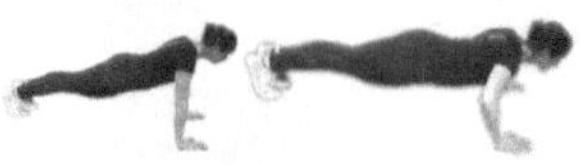

### 2 glute bridges

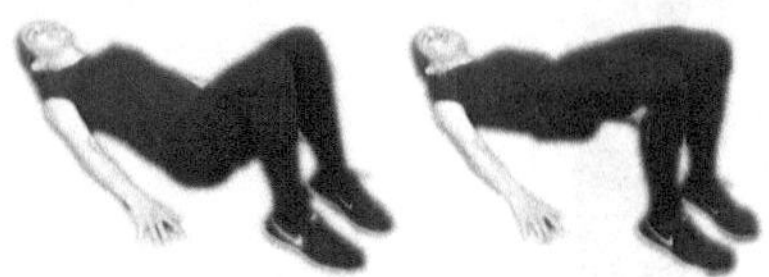

### 3 walking lunges x40

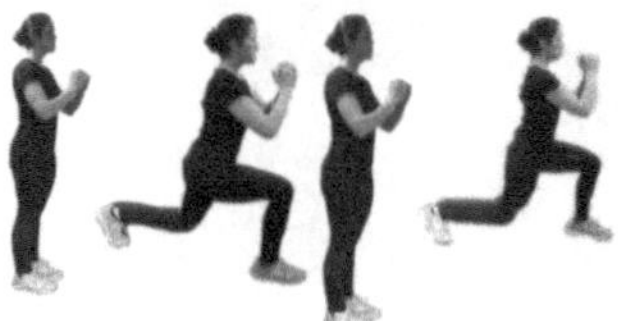

### 4 half burpee

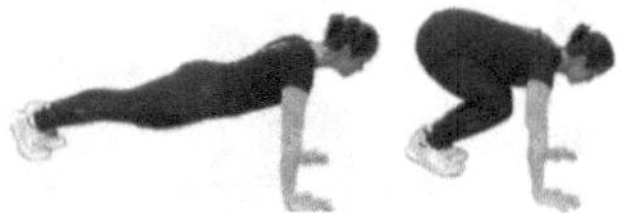

### 5 oblique twist

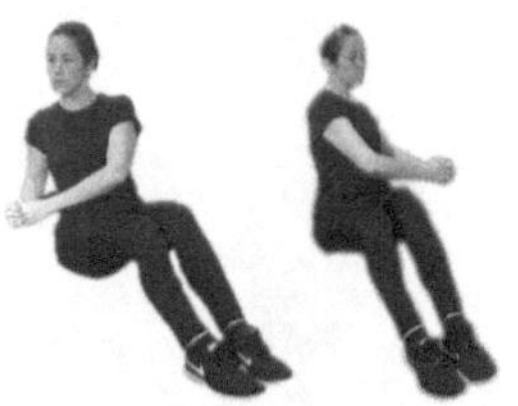

### 6 high knees

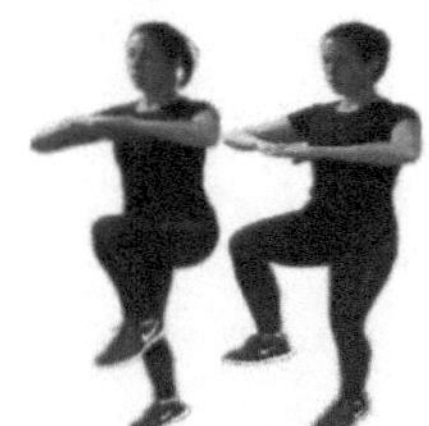

### 7 jumping jacks x50

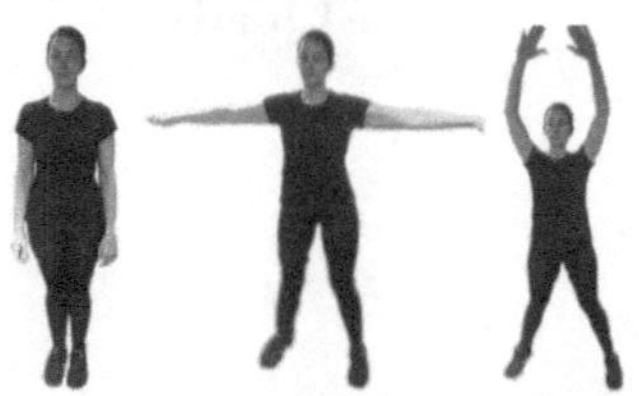

## Rest period between circuit rounds 2 min then begin circuits again.

## Cool down – 10 min- see page

Thursday Cardio & flexibility training
Week 1 pre-training

**2 x 5** min
warmup & cool down

**30** min
workout time

**40** min
total time

## Warm up -5 min

## Cardio - 30 min

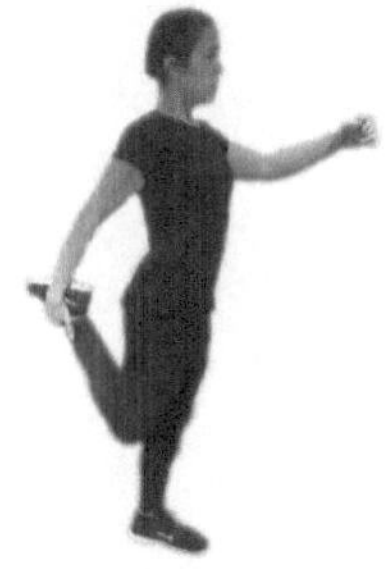

Quad stretch

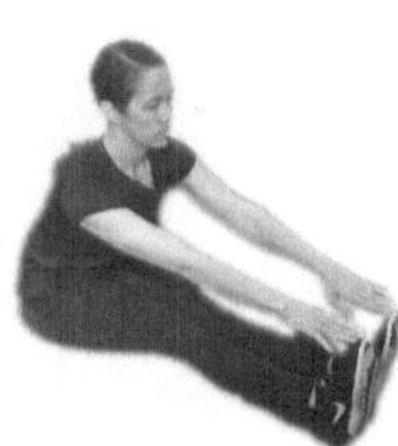

Hamstring stretch

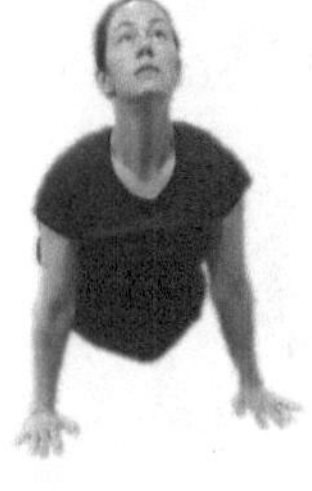

Abdominals

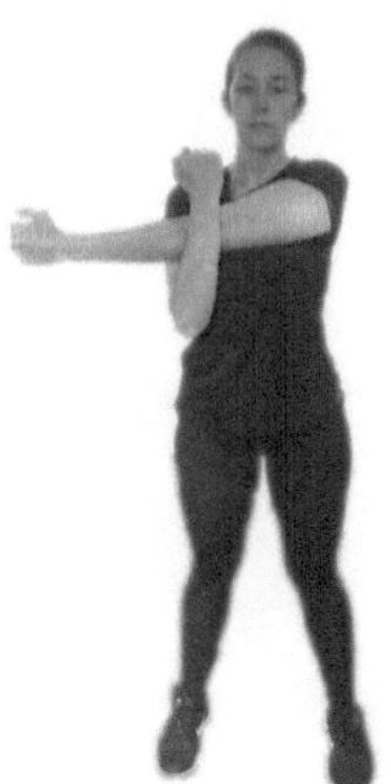

Upper back stretch

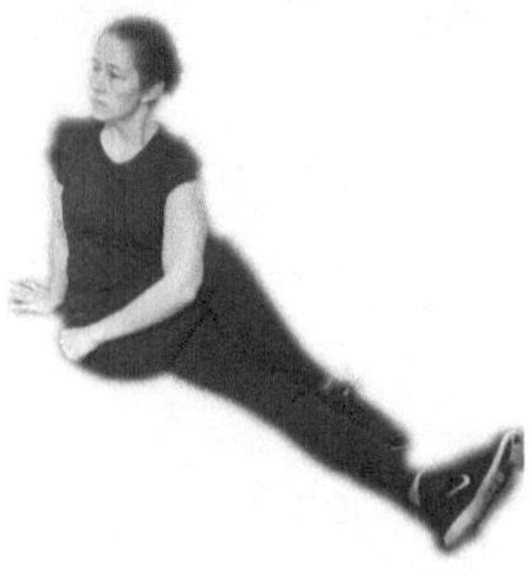

Rotational

## Make sure to follow stretches on page

## Cool down – 5 min- see page

Friday Pioneer Power Training workout
Week 1 pre-training

**1 x 6** min
circuits

**6** min
workout time

**26** min
total time

## Warm up -10 min

## F.H.I.T Circuit - 7 min - Repeat 2 times

**1** Sumo Squats x12

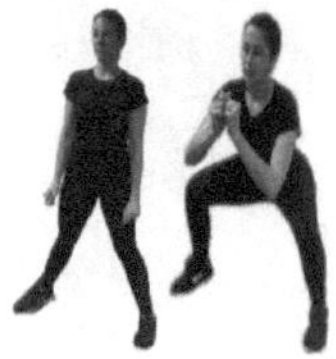

**3** Abdominal bicycles x12

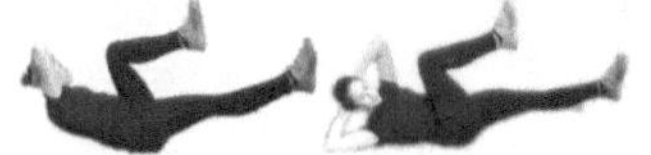

**2** Push up x12

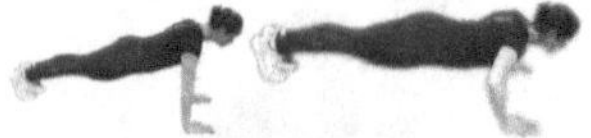

**4** High Knee 1min

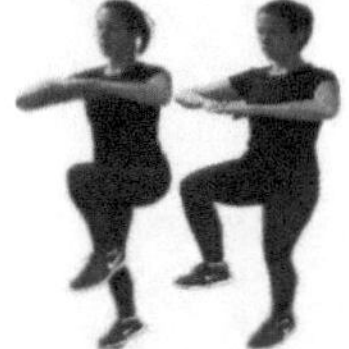

The 6minute clock is continuous. Continue to move through the circuit, performing the repetitions required.

Cool down – 10 min- see page

Monday Functional High Intensity Training workout

Week 2 pre-training

**2 x 7** min
circuits

**14** min
workout time

**37** min
total time

## Warm up -10 min

## F.H.I.T Circuit - 7 min - Repeat 2 times

1 walking lungex30

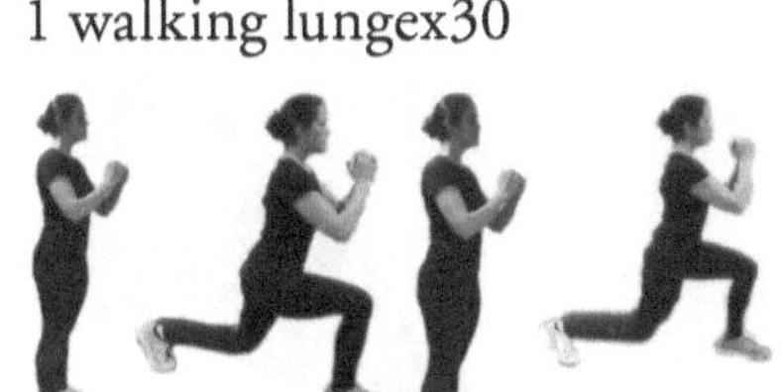

2 side shuffle 1min

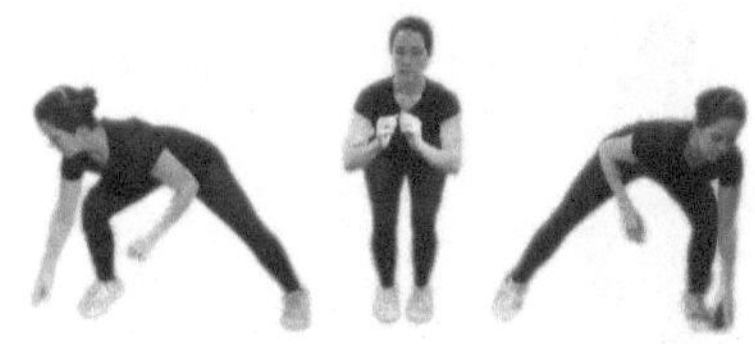

3 leg lifts x25

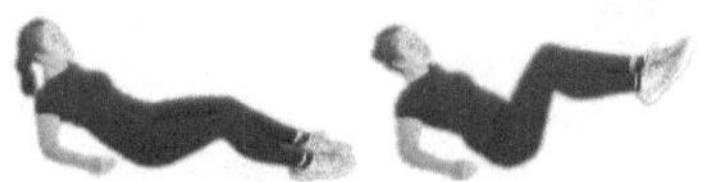

4 plank jacks x40

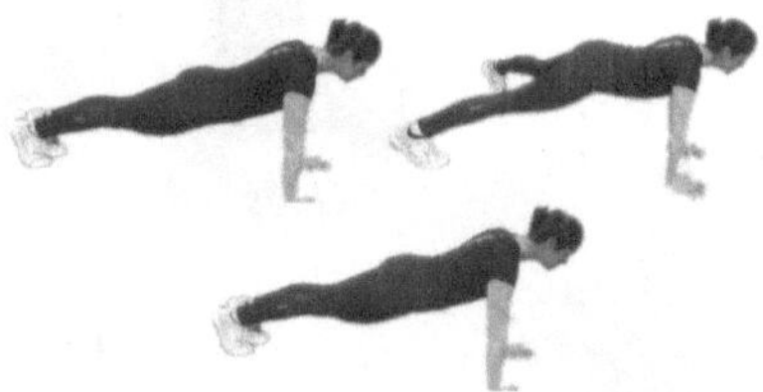

5 superman x25

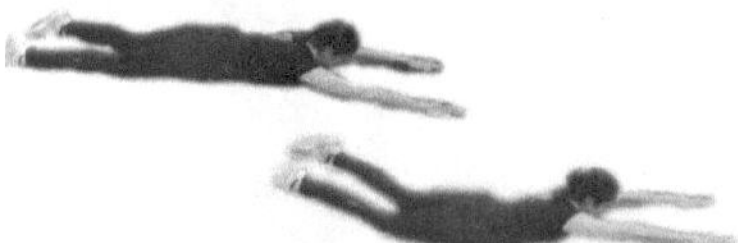

6 heel raises x30

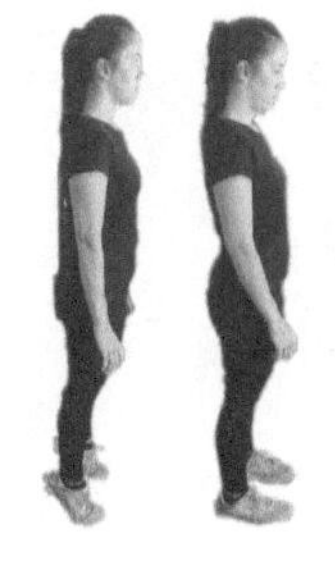

7 butt kicks 1 min

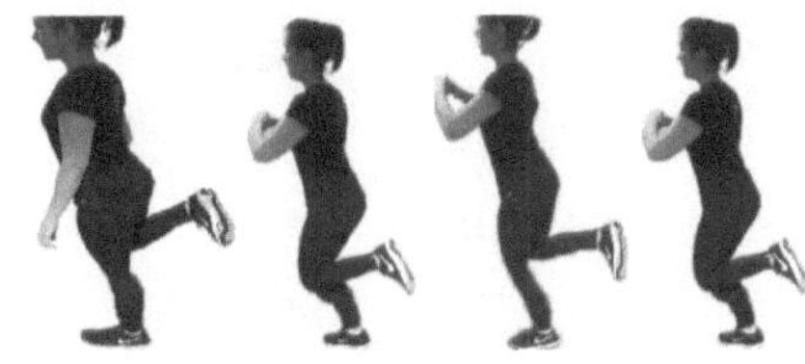

Rest period between circuit rounds 2 min then begin circuits again.

Cool down – 10 min- see page

Tuesday is recovery training

Week 2 pre-training

**2 x 5** min
warmup & cool down

**30** min
workout time

**40** min
total time

## Warm up -5 min

## Cardio - 30 min

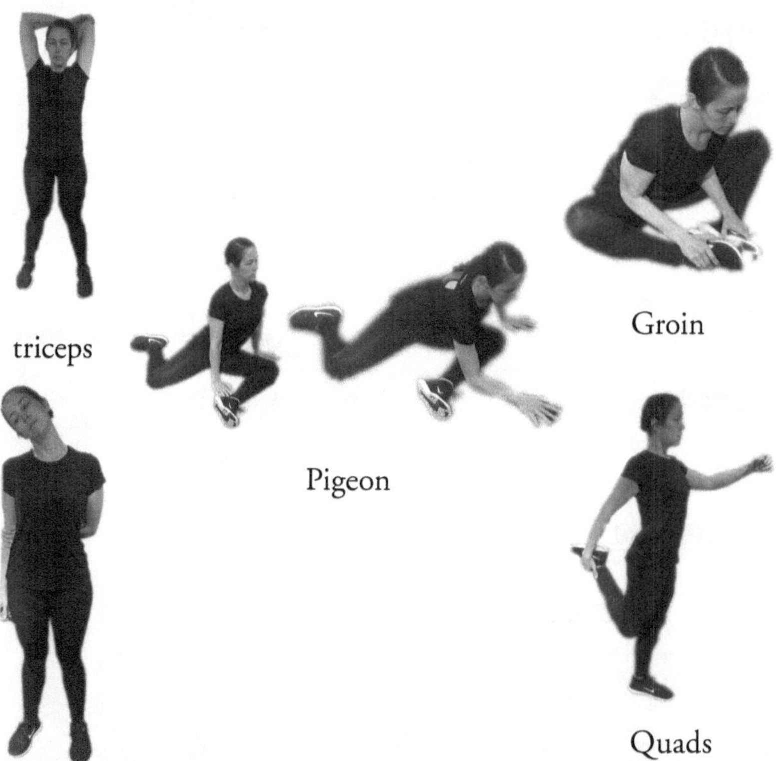



## Make sure to follow stretches on page

## Cool down – 5 min- see page

wednesday Functional High Intensity Training workout

Week 2 pre-training

**2 x 7** min
circuits

**14** min
workout time

**37** min
total time

## Warm up -10 min

## F.H.I.T Circuit - 7 min - Repeat 2 times

### 1 push up x30

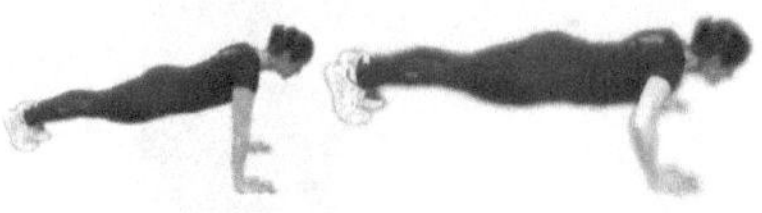

### 3 half burpee x25

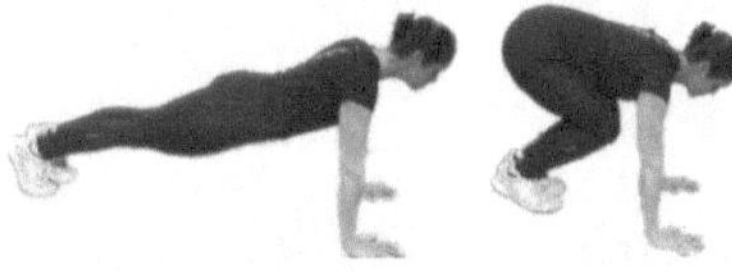

### 5 glute bridges x30

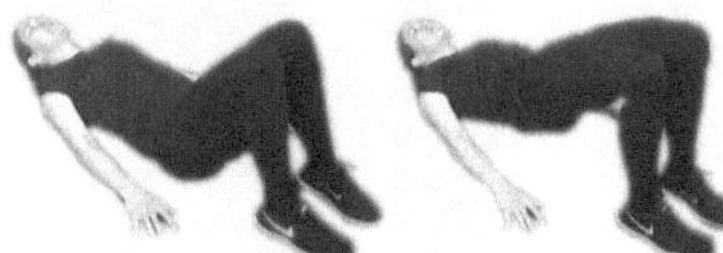

### 7 lateral shuffles 1 min

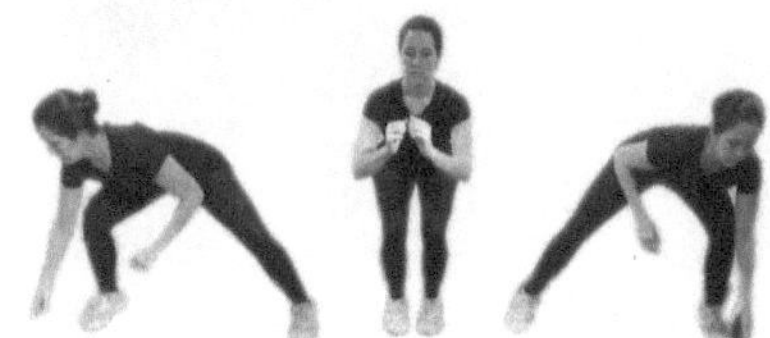

### 2 Alternating lateral lunge x20

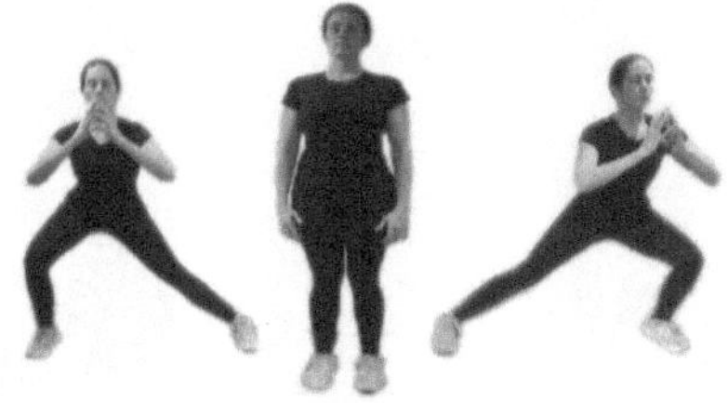

### 4 abdominal bicycles x40

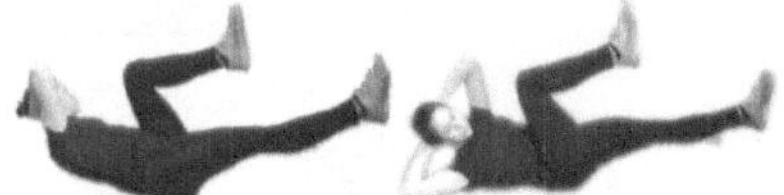

### 6 jumping jacks x50

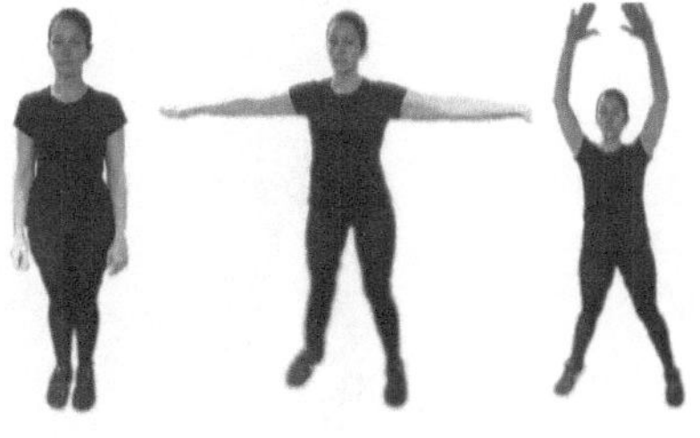

## Rest period between circuit rounds 2 min then begin circuits again.

## Cool down – 10 min- see page

Thursday Cardio & flexibility training
Week 2 pre-training

**2 x 5** min
warmup & cool down

**30**min
workout time

**40**min
total time

## Warm up -5 min

## Cardio - 30 min

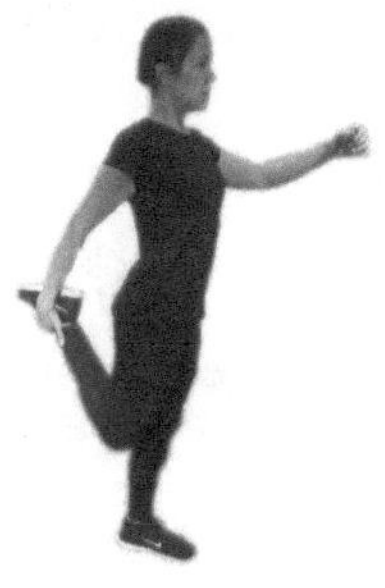

Quad stretch

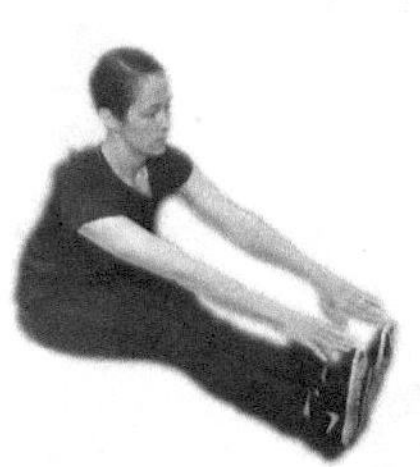

Hamstring stretch

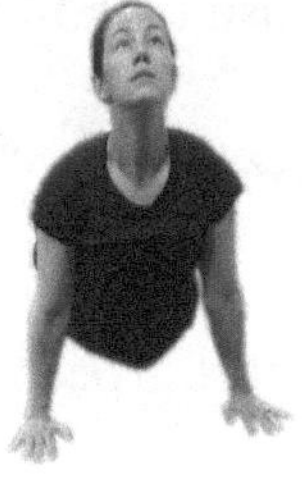

Abdominals

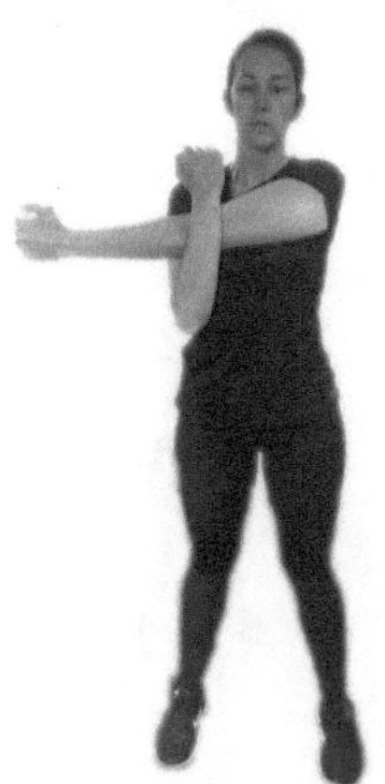

Upper back stretch

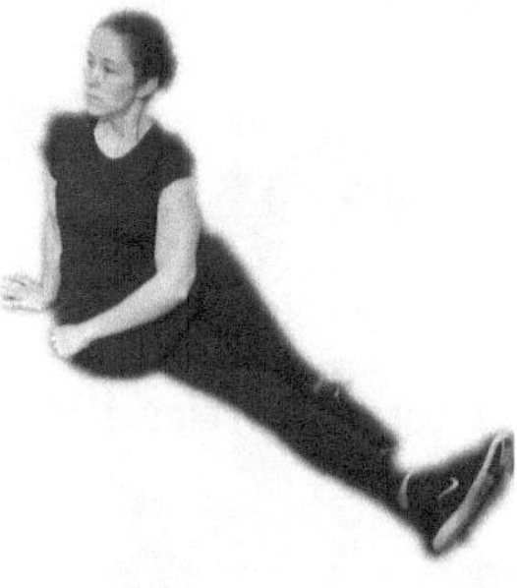

Rotational

## Make sure to follow stretches on page

## Cool down – 5 min- see page

Friday Pioneer Power Training
workout

**1 x 6** min circuits  **6** min workout time  **26** min total time

Week 2 pre-training

## Warm up -10 min

## F.H.I.T Circuit - 7 min - Repeat 2 times

**1** Alternating lateral lunge x12

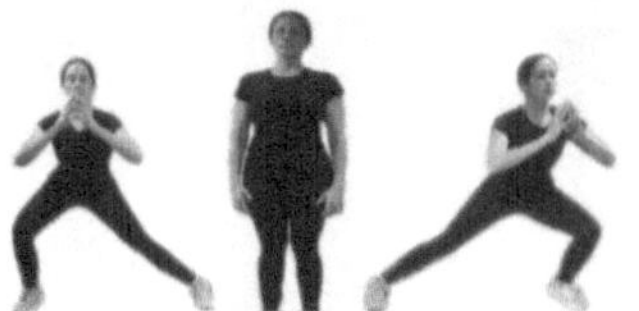

**2** Half Burpees x12

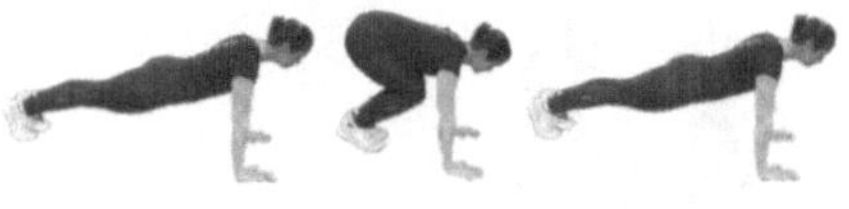

**4** High Knee 1min

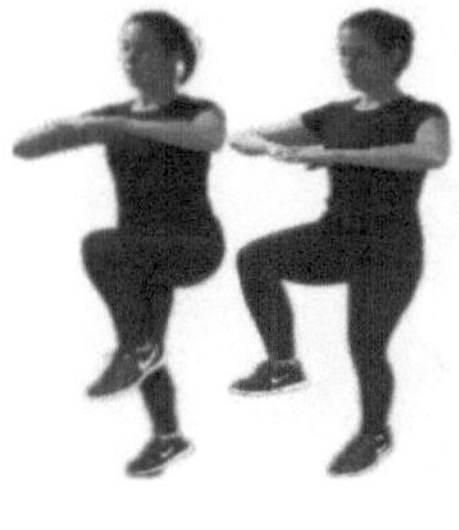

**3** Seated Russian twist x12

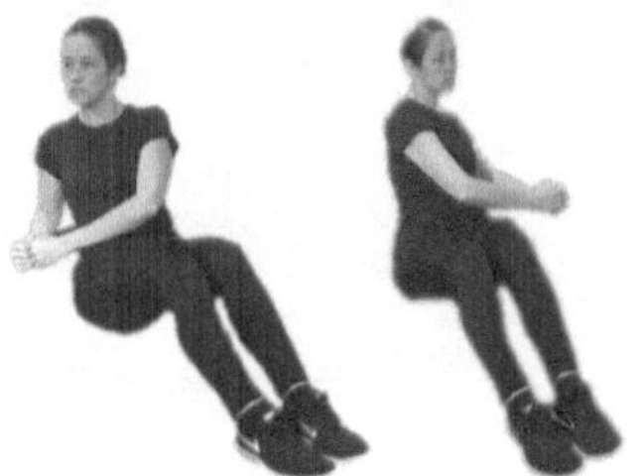

The 6minute clock is continuous. Continue to move through the circuit, performing the repetitions required.

Cool down – 10 min- see page

Monday Functional High
Intensity Training workout
Week 3 pre-training

**2 x 7** min
circuits

**14** min
workout time

**37** min
total time

## Warm up -10 min

## F.H.I.T Circuit - 7 min - Repeat 2 times

1 sumo squat x30

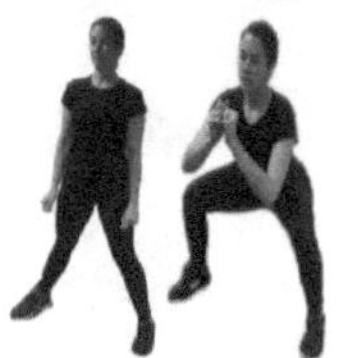

2 high knees 1min

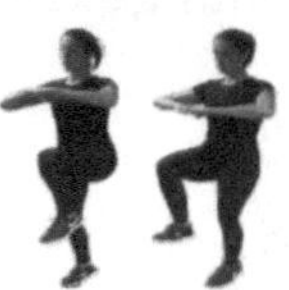

3 leg scissors x25

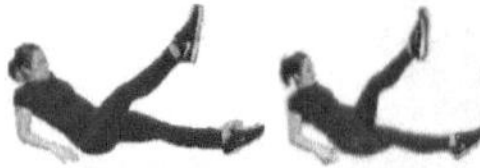

4 butt kicks x1m

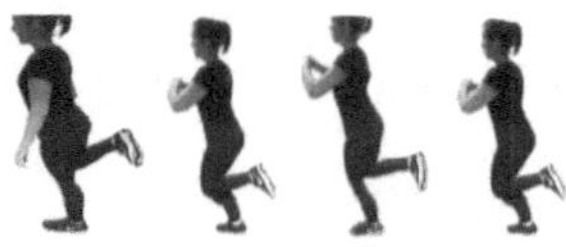

5 Triceps dips x25

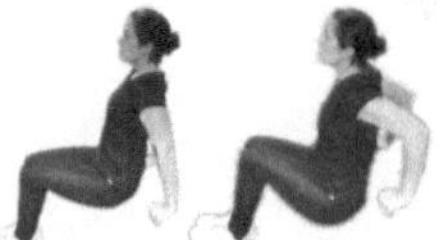

6 Ab bicycle x30

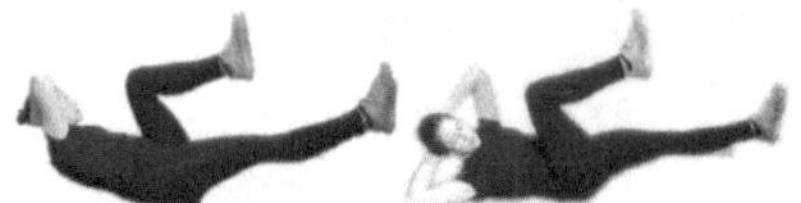

7 side shuffles 1min

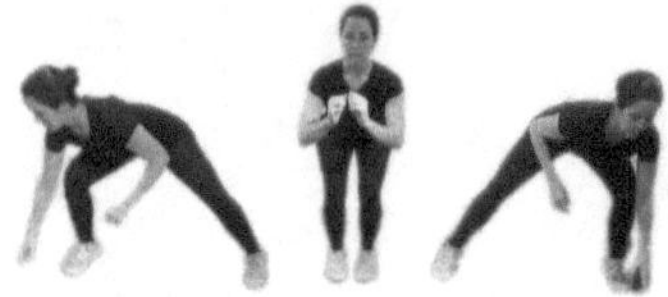

Rest period between circuit rounds 2 min then begin circuits again.

Cool down – 10 min- see page

Tuesday is recovery training

Week 3 pre-training

**2 x 5** min
warmup & cool down

**30** min
workout time

**40** min
total time

## Warm up -5 min

## Cardio - 30 min

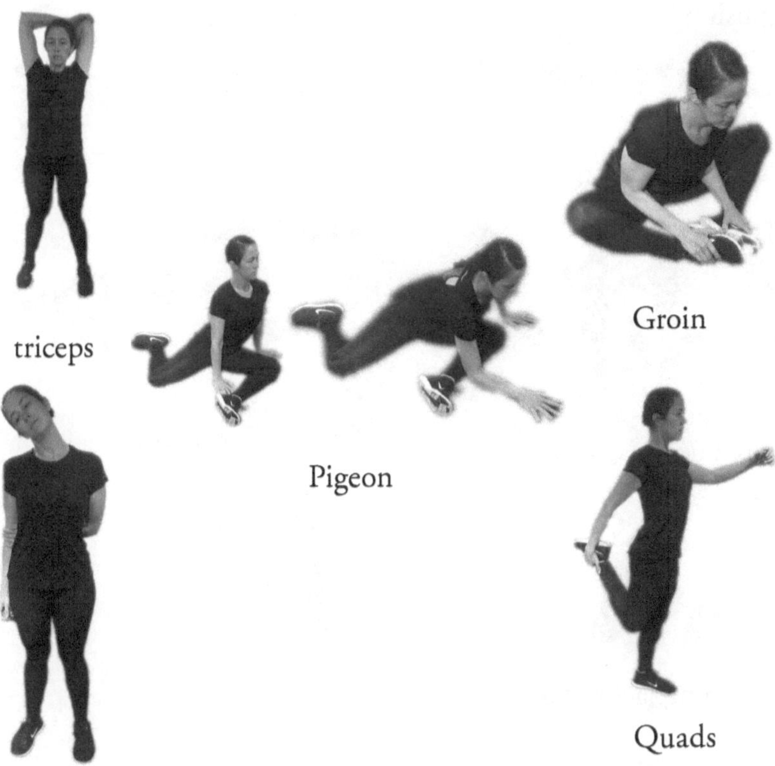


## Make sure to follow stretches on page

## Cool down – 5 min- see page

wednesday Functional High Intensity Training workout

Week 3 pre-training

**2 x 7** min
circuits

**14** min
workout time

**37** min
total time

## Warm up -10 min

## F.H.I.T Circuit - 7 min - Repeat 2 times

### 1 push up x30

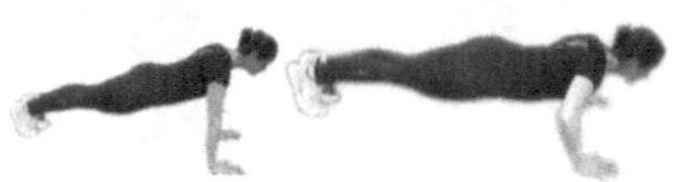

### 2 Glute Bridges x30

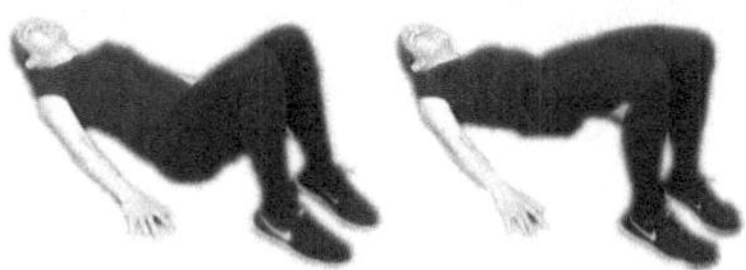

### 3 Walking lunges x24

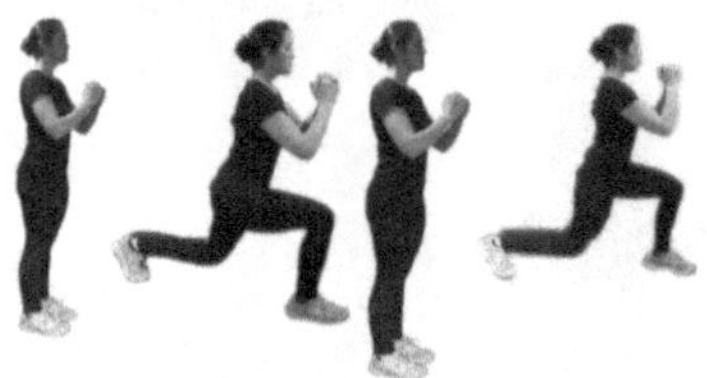

### 4 half burpee x20

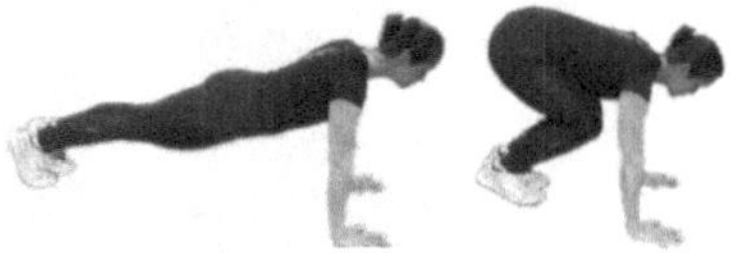

### 5 oblique twist x40

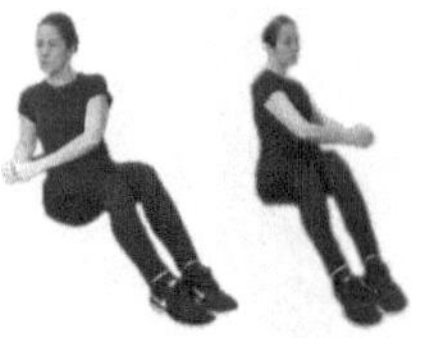

### 6 high knee x1min

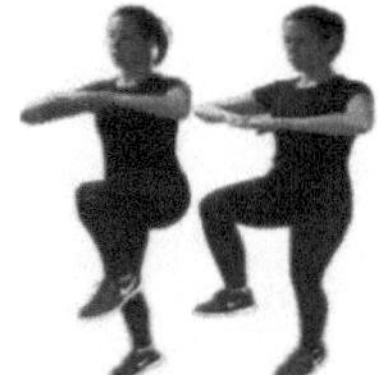

### 7 jumping jacks x50

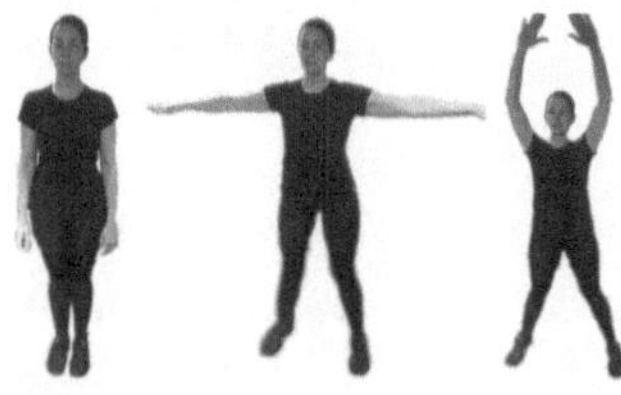

Rest period between circuit rounds 2 min then begin circuits again.

Cool down – 10 min- see page

Thursday Cardio & flexibility training
Week 3 pre-training

**2 x 5** min
warmup & cool down

**30** min
workout time

**40** min
total time

## Warm up -5 min

## Cardio - 30 min

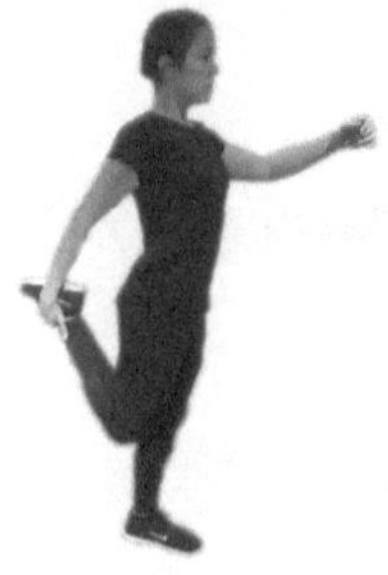

Quad stretch

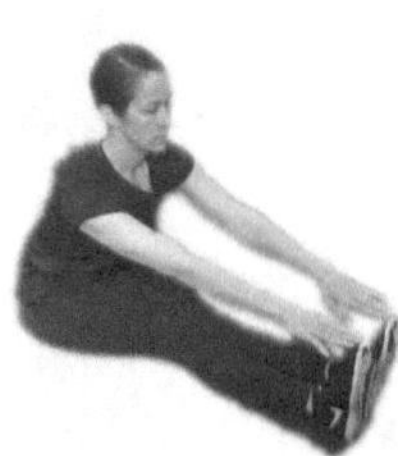

Hamstring stretch

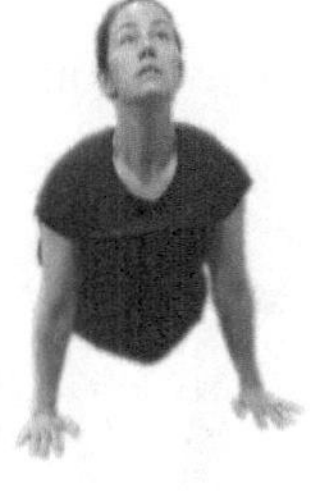

Abdominals

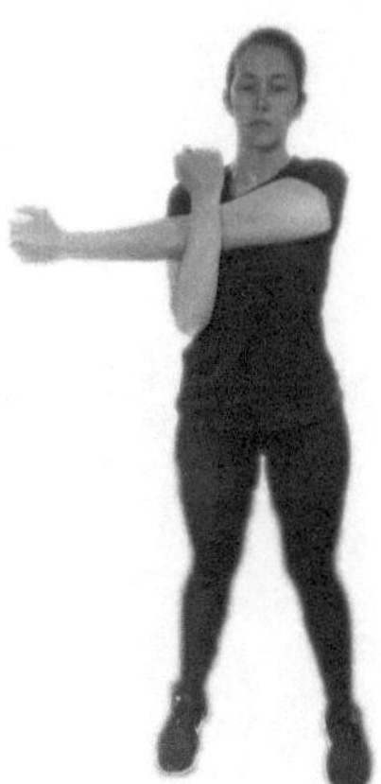

Upper back stretch

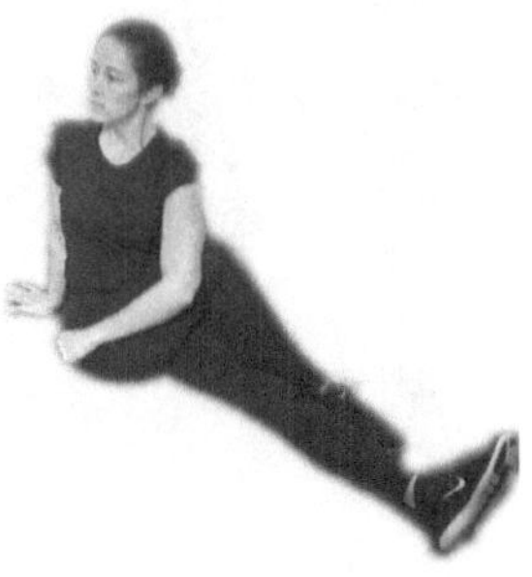

Rotational

## Make sure to follow stretches on page

## Cool down – 5 min- see page

Friday Pioneer Power Training workout
Week 3 pre-training

**1 x 6**min
circuits

**6**min
workout time

**26**min
total time

## Warm up -10 min

## F.H.I.T Circuit - 7 min - Repeat 2 times

① sumo squat jump x12

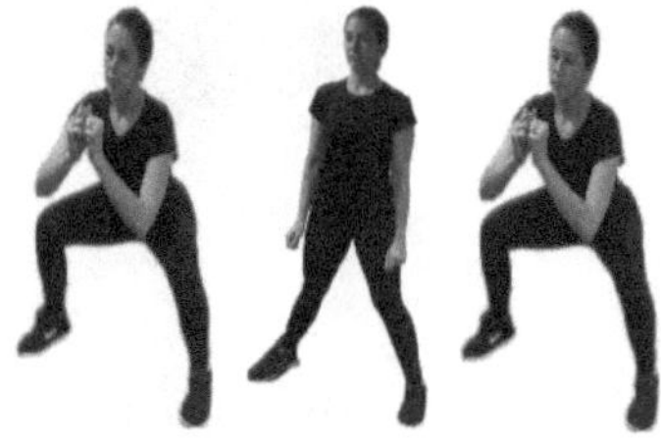

② Push x12

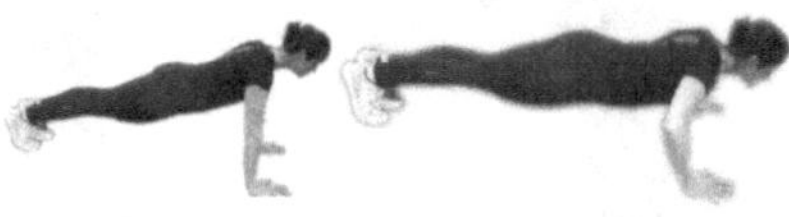

④ ab bicycles x12

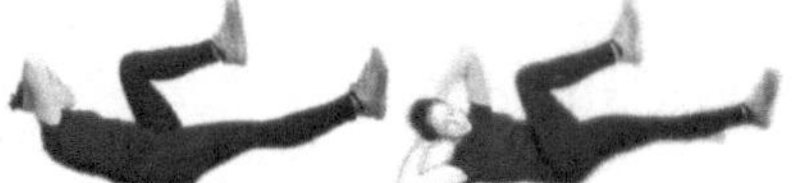

③ high knees 1min

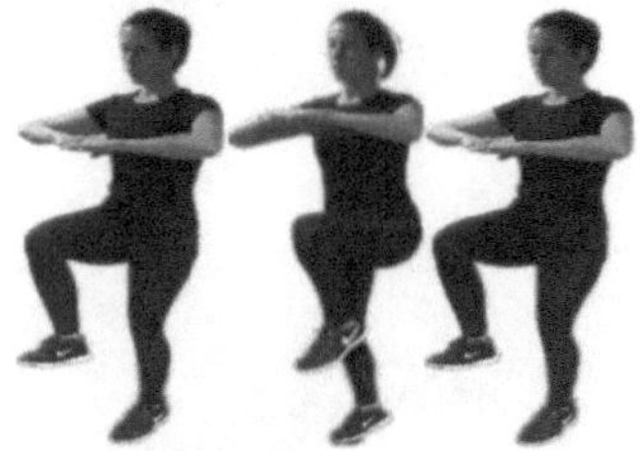

The 6minute clock is continuous. Continue to move through the circuit, performing the repetitions required.

## Cool down – 10 min- see page

Monday Functional High
Intensity Training workout

Week 4 pre-training

**2 x 7** min
circuits

**14**min
workout time

**37**min
total time

## Warm up -10 min

## F.H.I.T Circuit - 7 min - Repeat 2 times

1 walking lunge x30

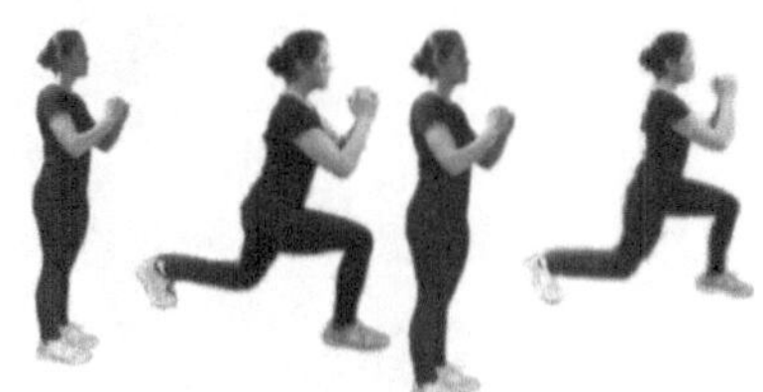

2 side shuffle 1min

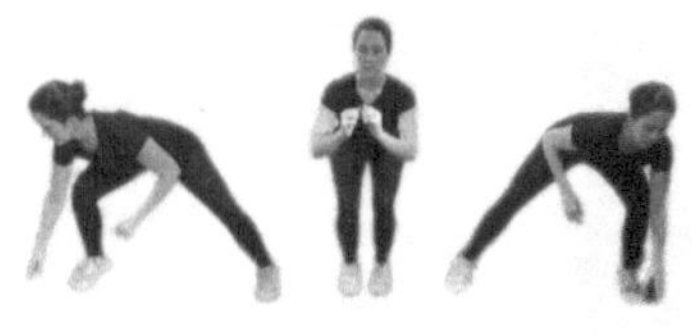

4 plank jacks x1m

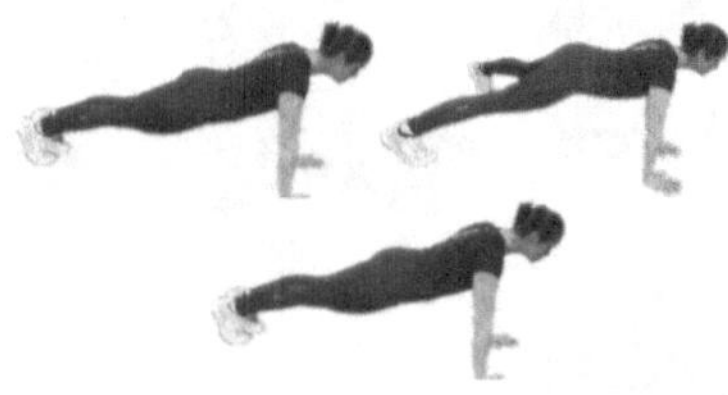

3 leg lifts x25

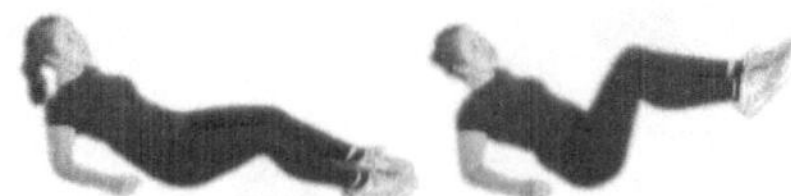

5 superman x25

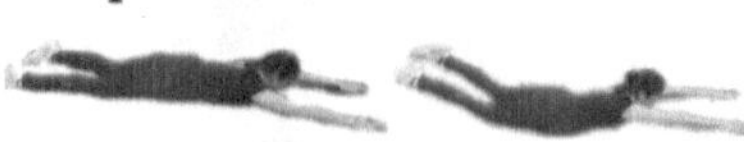

6 heel raise x30

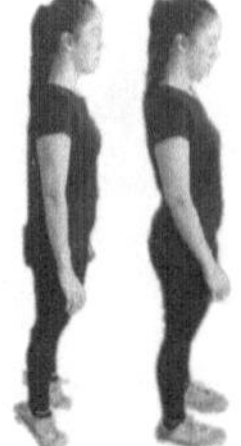

7 butt kicks 1min

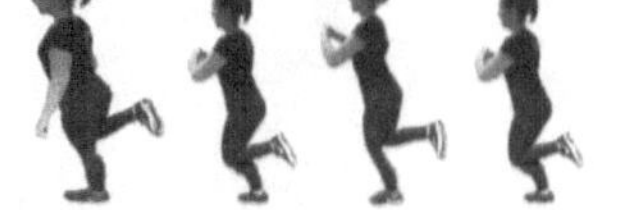

## Rest period between circuit rounds 2 min then begin circuits again.

## Cool down – 10 min- see page

Tuesday is recovery training

Week 4 pre-training

**2 x 5** min
warmup & cool down

**30** min
workout time

**40** min
total time

## Warm up -5 min

## Cardio - 30 min

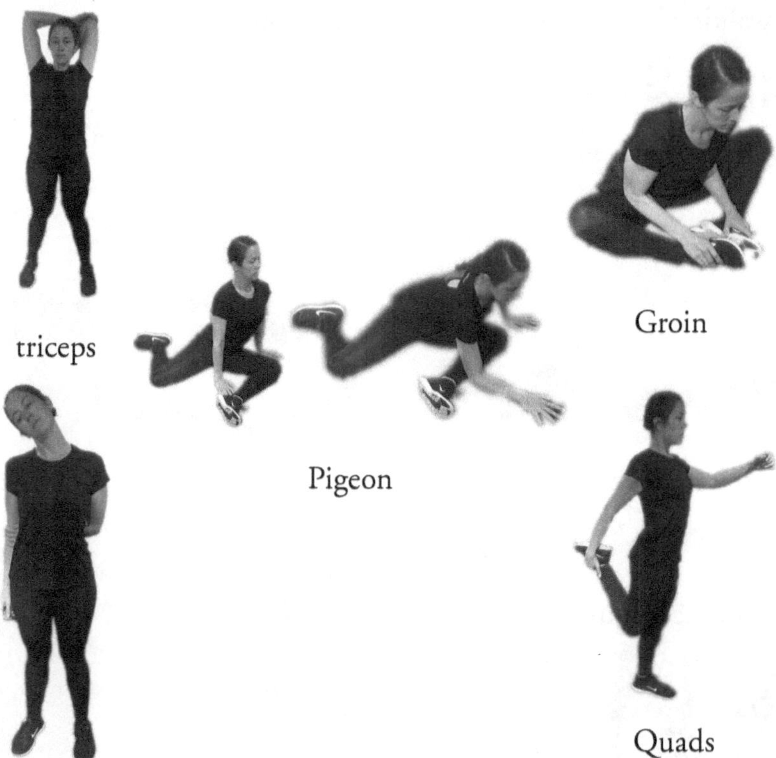


Make sure to follow stretches on page

Cool down – 5 min- see page

wednesday Functional High
Intensity Training workout
Week 4 pre-training

**2 x 7** min
circuits

**14**min
workout time

**37**min
total time

## Warm up -10 min

## F.H.I.T Circuit - 7 min - Repeat 2 times

1 push up x30

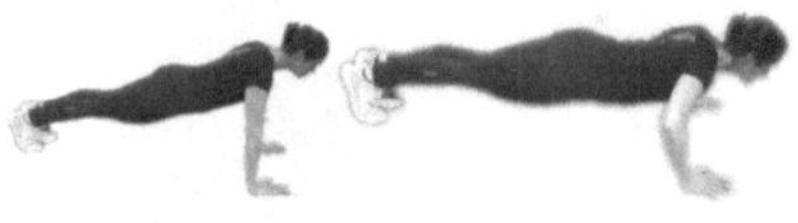

2 alternating side lunge x30

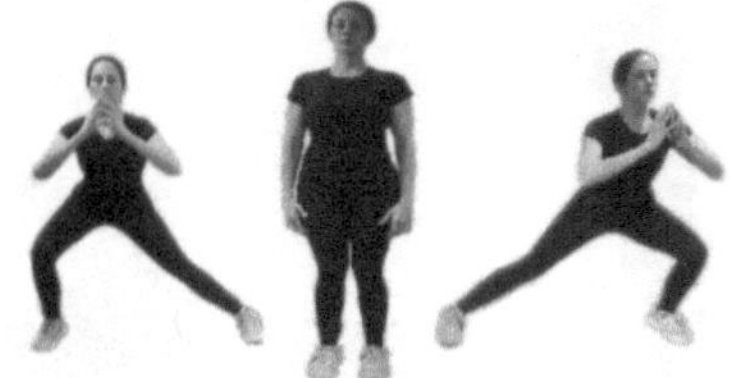

3 half burpees x25

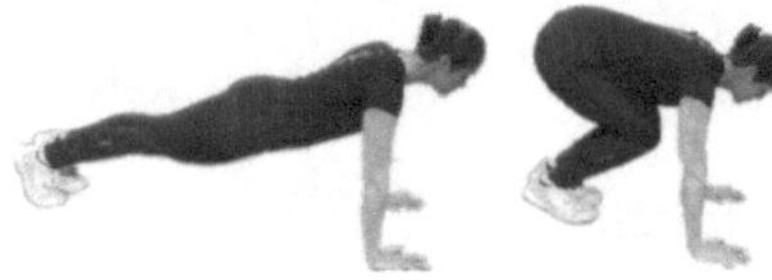

4 AB bicycle x40

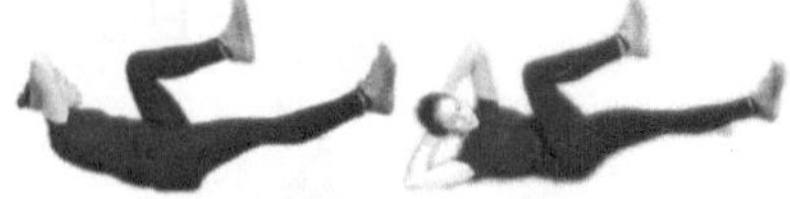

5 glute bridges x30

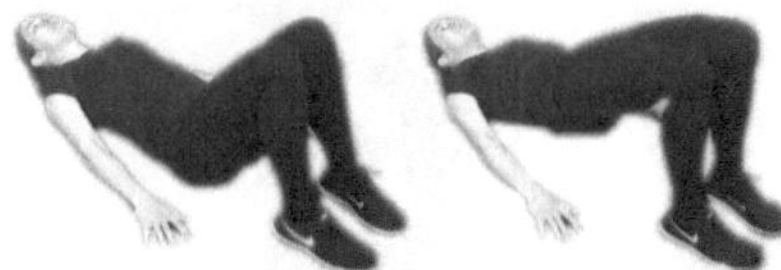

6 jumping jacks x1min

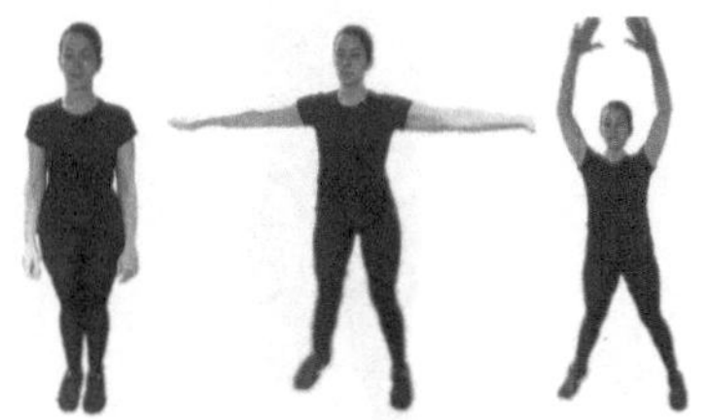

7 lateral shuffle 1min

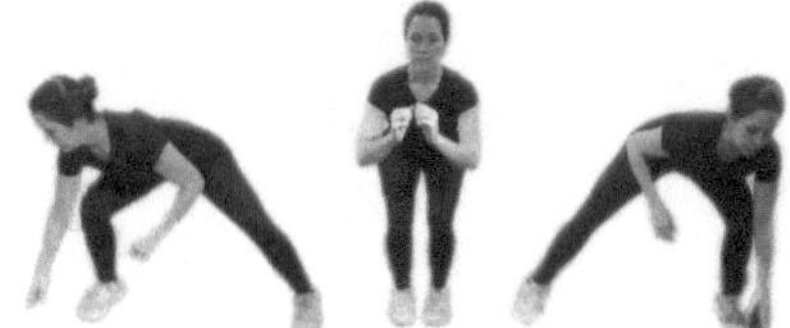

Rest period between circuit rounds 2 min then begin circuits again.

Cool down – 10 min- see page

Thursday Cardio & flexibility training
Week 4 pre-training

**2 x 5** min
warmup & cool down

**30** min
workout time

**40** min
total time

## Warm up -5 min

## Cardio - 30 min

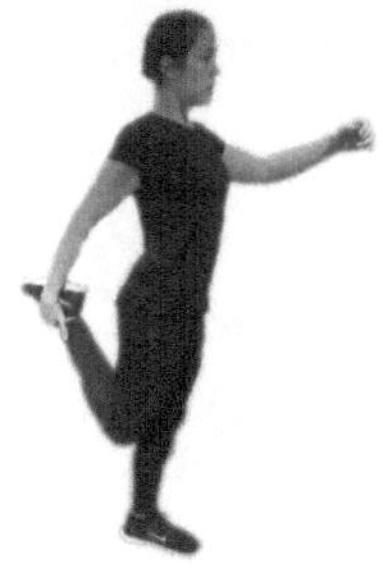

Quad stretch

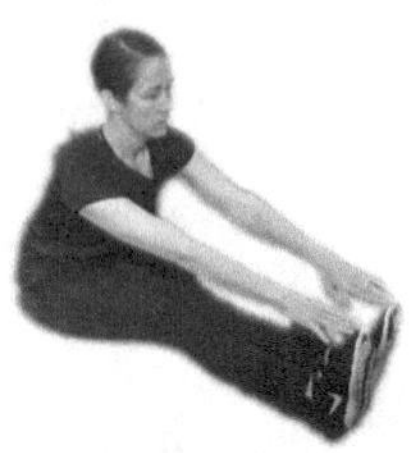

Hamstring stretch

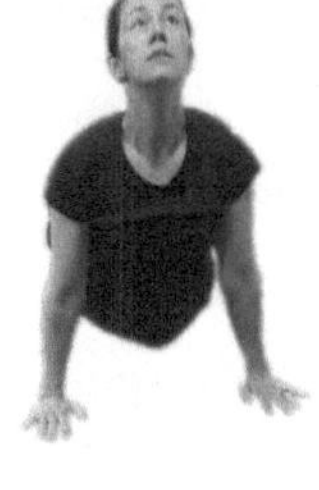

Abdominals

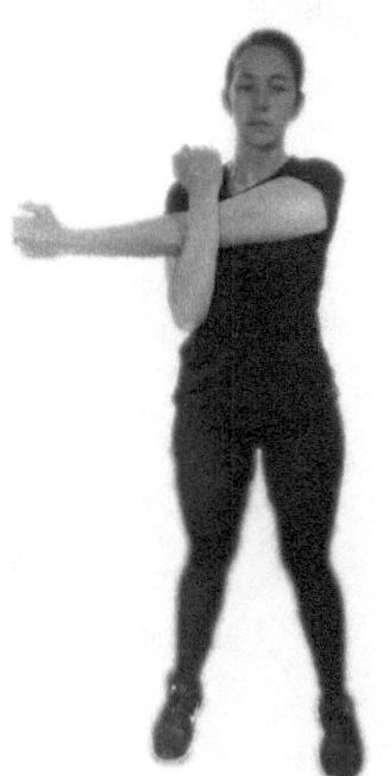

Upper back stretch

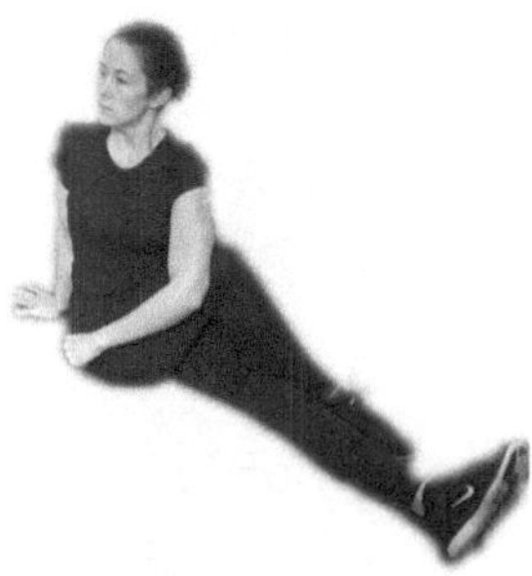

Rotational

## Make sure to follow stretches on page

## Cool down – 5 min- see page

Friday Pioneer Power Training workout
Week 4 pre-training

**1 x 6**min
circuits

**6**min
workout time

**26**min
total time

## Warm up -10 min

## F.H.I.T Circuit - 7 min - Repeat 2 times

1  alternating lateral lunges x12

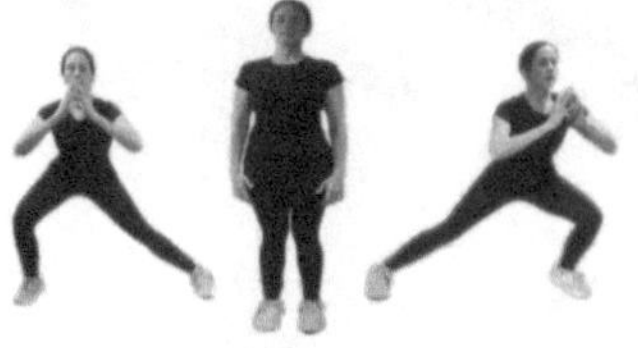

3  high knees 1min

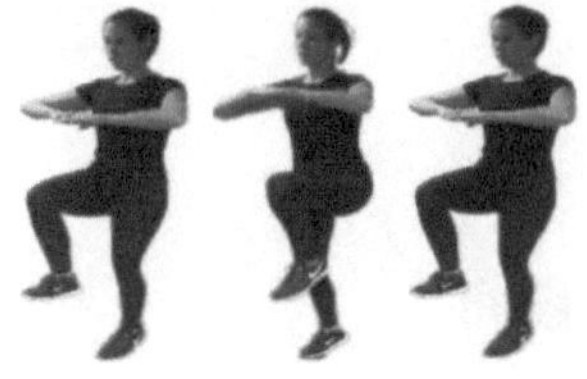

2  half burpees x12

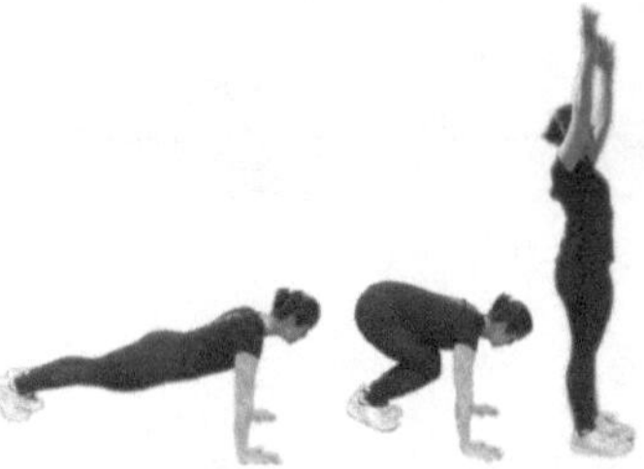

4  seated Russian twist x12

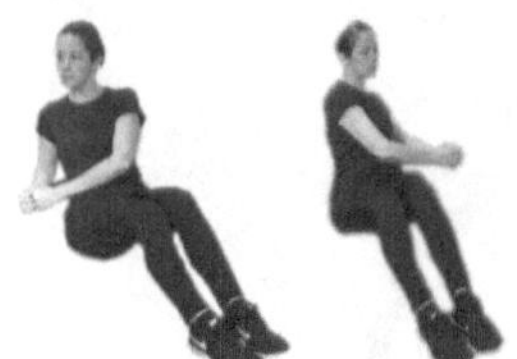

The 6minute clock is continuous. Continue to move through the circuit, performing the repetitions required.

Cool down – 10 min- see page

Monday Functional High
Intensity Training workout
Week 1

**2 x 7** min
circuits

**14** min
workout time

**37** min
total time

## Warm up -10 min

## F.H.I.T Circuit - 7 min - Repeat 2 times

1 pioneer pulse squats

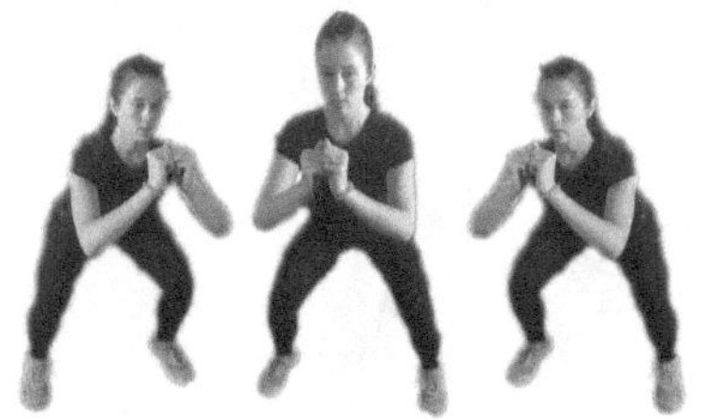

3 Squat jump

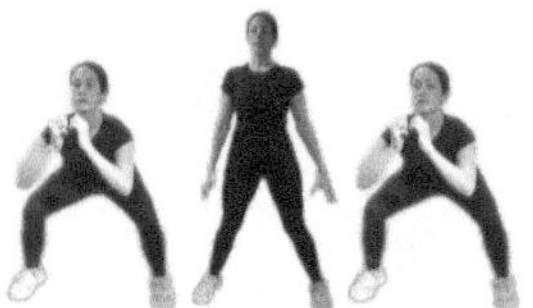

5 high knee

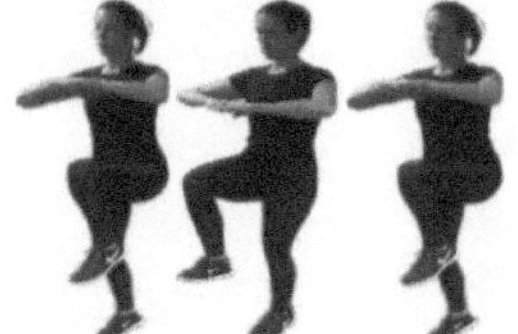

7 knee pulls

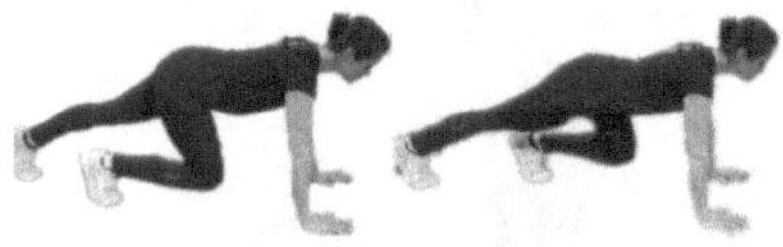

2 push ups

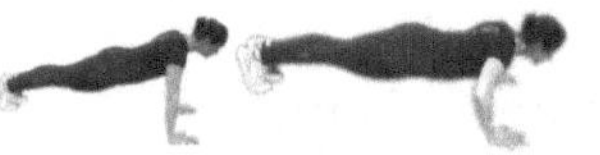

4 bench dips

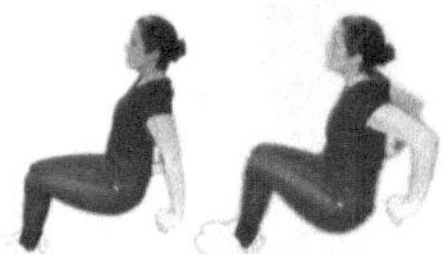

6 bicycles

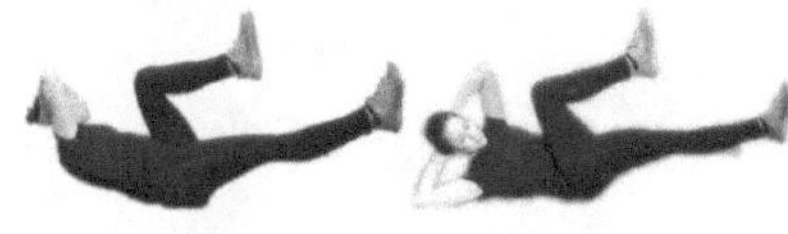

Rest period between circuit rounds 2 min then begin circuits again.

Cool down – 10 min- see page

Tuesday is recovery training

Week 1 pre-training

**2 x 5**<sub>min</sub> warmup & cool down

**30**<sub>min</sub> workout time

**40**<sub>min</sub> total time

## Warm up -5 min

## Cardio - 30 min

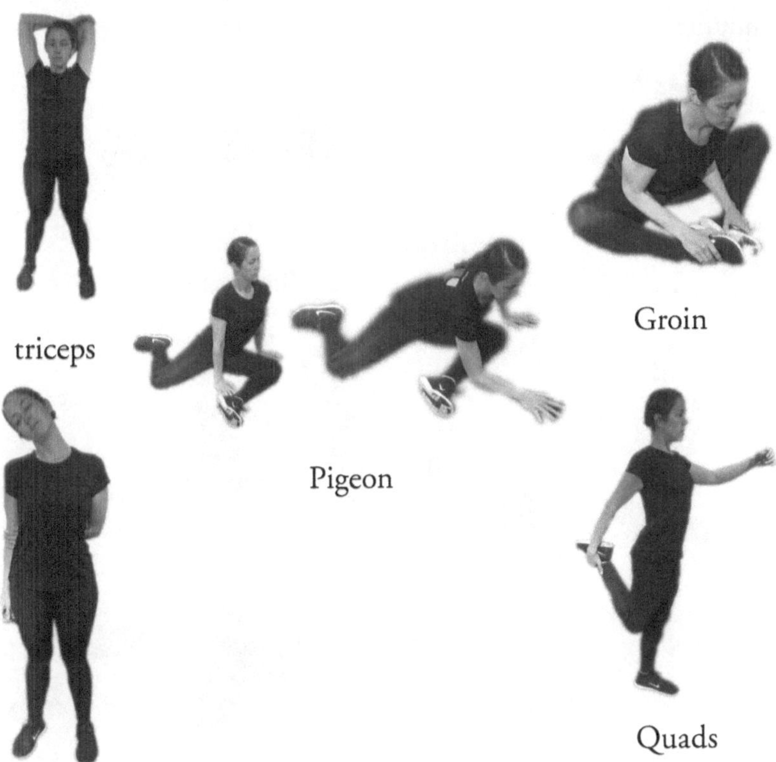



Make sure to follow stretches on page

Cool down – 5 min- see page

Wednesday Functional High
Intensity Training workout
Week 1

**2 x 7** min
circuits

**14** min
workout time

**37** min
total time

## Warm up -10 min

## F.H.I.T Circuit - 7 min - Repeat 2 times

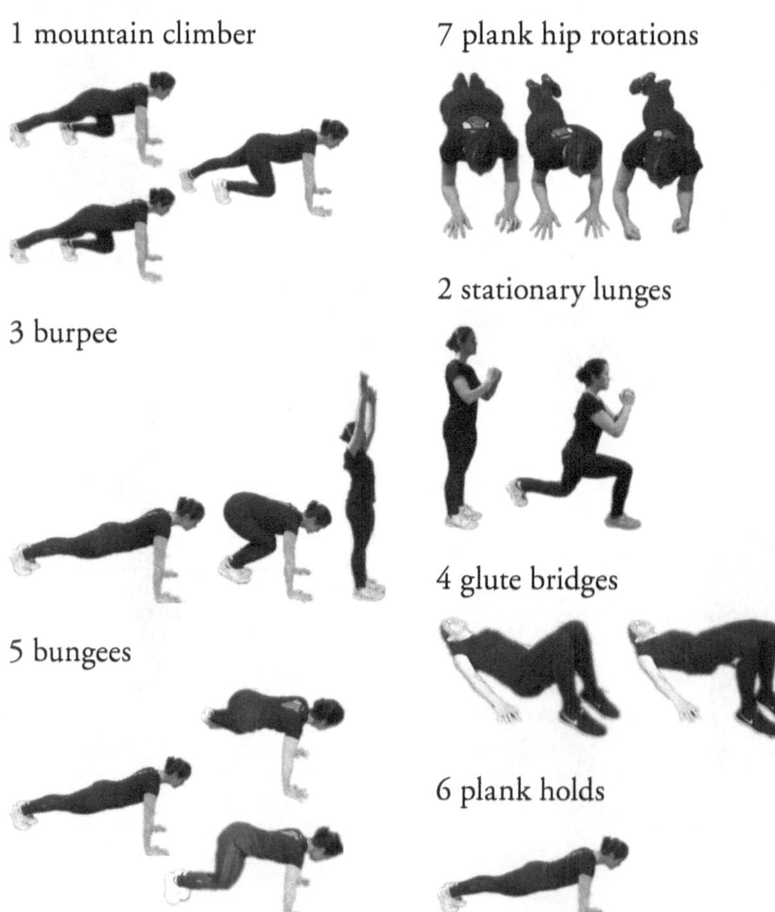

1 mountain climber

7 plank hip rotations

2 stationary lunges

3 burpee

4 glute bridges

5 bungees

6 plank holds

Rest period between circuit rounds 2 min then begin circuits again.

Cool down – 10 min- see page

Thursday Cardio & flexibility training
Week 1 pre-training

**2 x 5** min
warmup & cool down

**30** min
workout time

**40** min
total time

## Warm up -5 min

## Cardio - 30 min

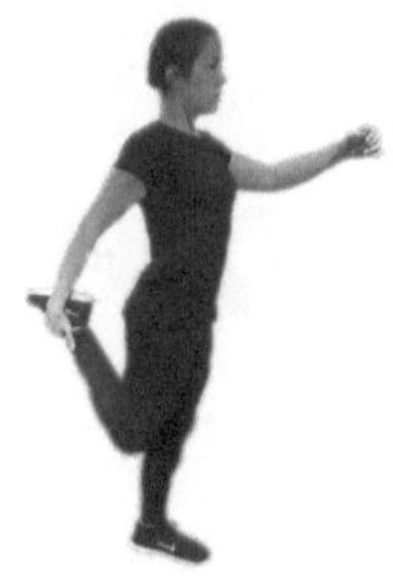

Quad stretch

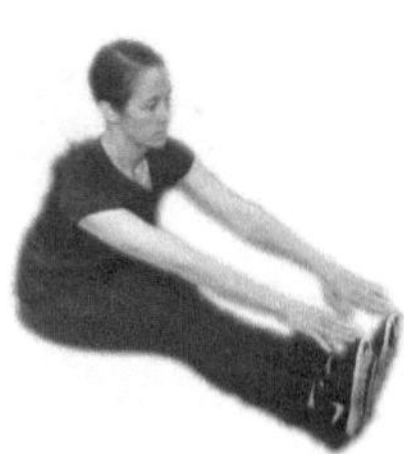

Hamstring stretch

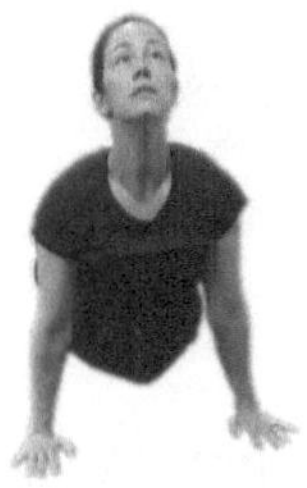

Abdominals

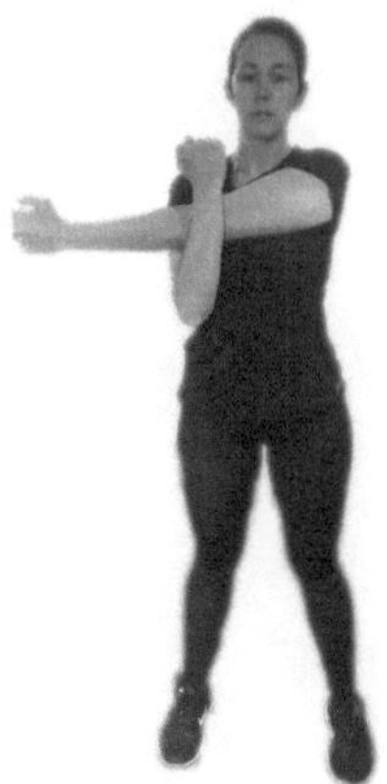

Upper back stretch

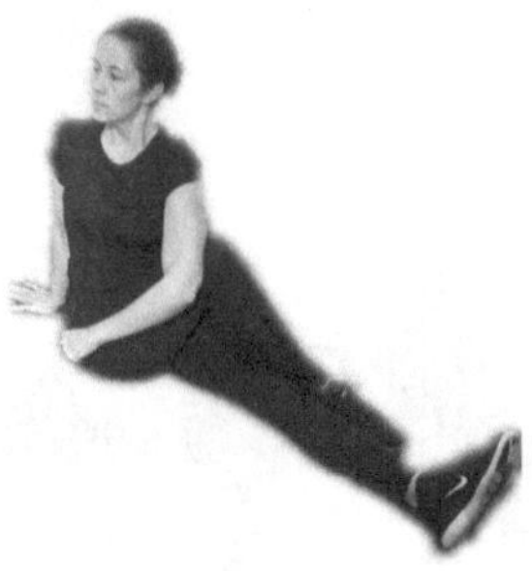

Rotational

## Make sure to follow stretches on page

## Cool down – 5 min- see page

Friday Pioneer Power Training
workout
Week 1

# 1 x 6 min
circuits

# 6 min
workout time

# 26 min
total time

## Warm up -10 min

## F.H.I.T Circuit - 7 min - Repeat 2 times

① push up incline x12

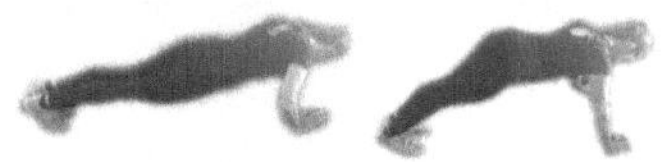

④ bicycles

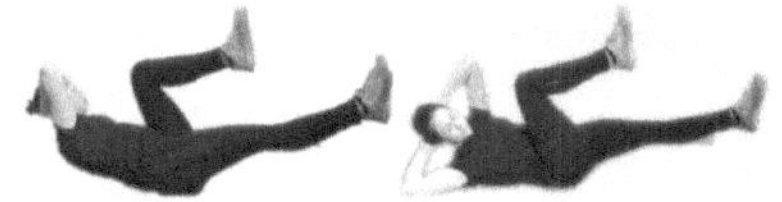

③ pioneer squats in and out

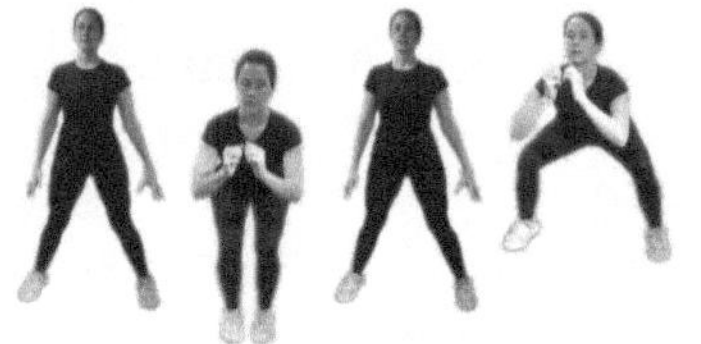

② 123 knee 1min

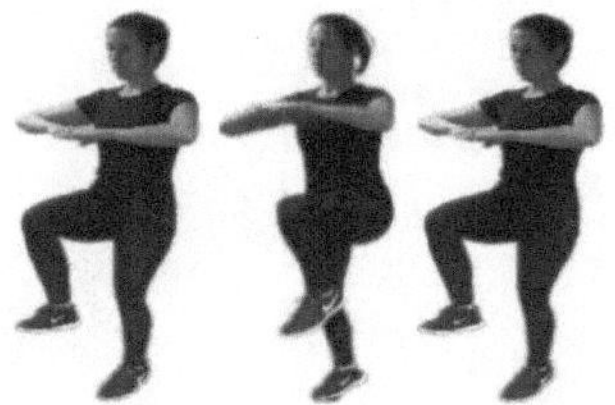

The 6minute clock is continuous. Continue to move through the circuit, performing the repetitions required.

## Cool down – 10 min- see page

Monday Functional High Intensity Training workout
Week 2

**2 x 7** min
circuits

**14** min
workout time

**37** min
total time

## Warm up -10 min

## F.H.I.T Circuit - 7 min - Repeat 2 times

1 lateral shuffle

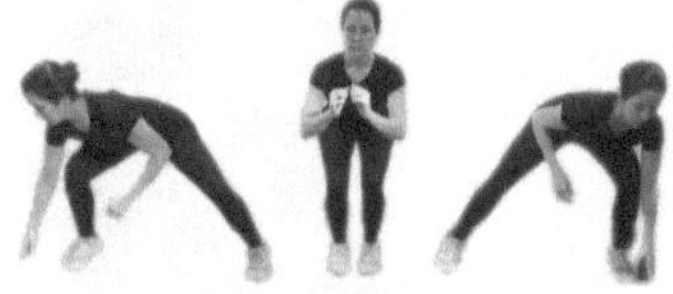

2 switch kicks

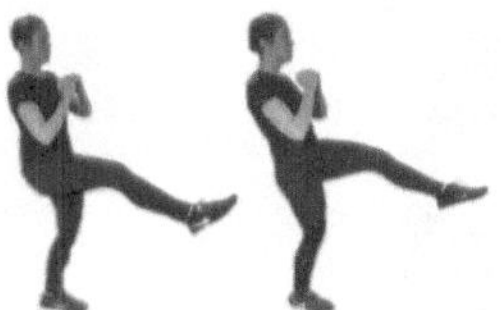

3 split jumps

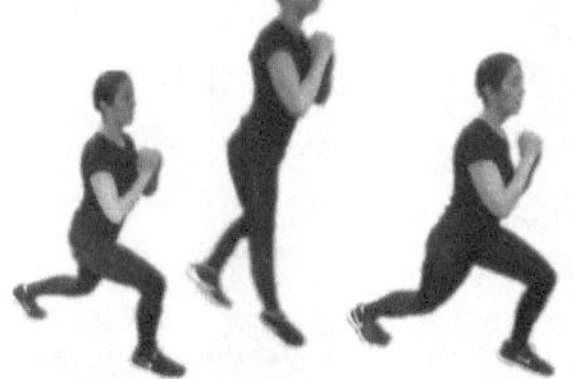

4 plank jacks

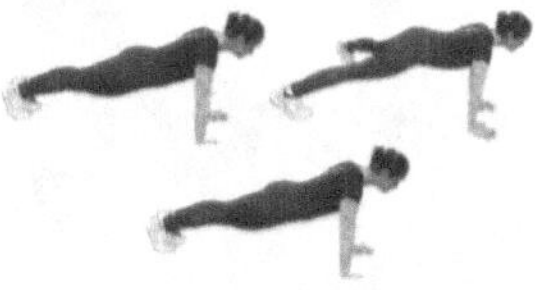

6 squat touch turn

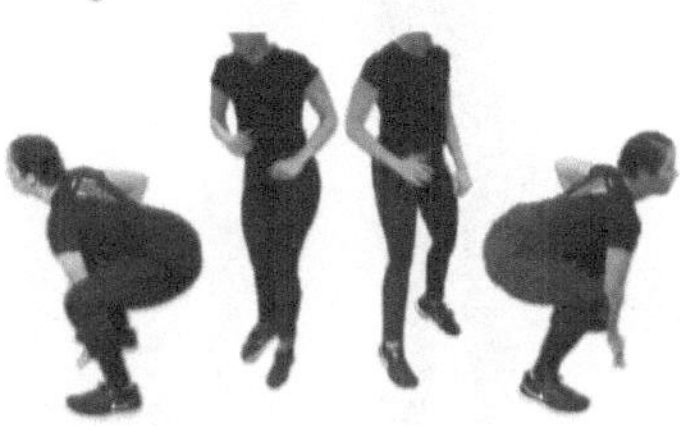

5 two push and move to left then to right

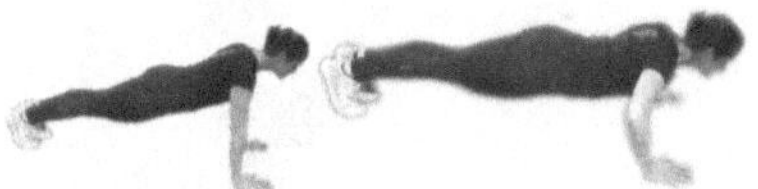

7 robot pushups

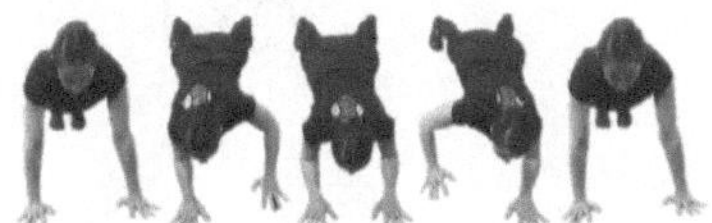

Rest period between circuit rounds 2 min then begin circuits again.

Cool down – 10 min- see page

Tuesday is recovery training

Week 2 pre-training

**2 x 5** min
warmup & cool down

**30**min
workout time

**40**min
total time

## Warm up -5 min

## Cardio - 30 min

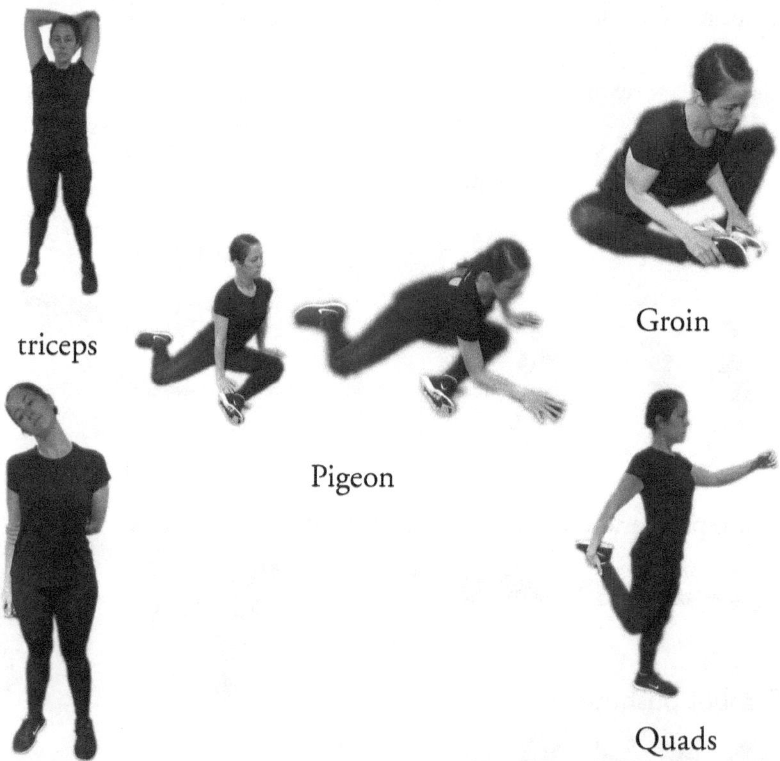

triceps

Groin

Pigeon

Neck & shoulder

Quads

Make sure to follow stretches on page

Cool down – 5 min- see page

Wednesday Functional High
Intensity Training workout
Week 2

**2 x 7** min
circuits

**14** min
workout time

**37** min
total time

## Warm up -10 min

## F.H.I.T Circuit - 7 min - Repeat 2 times

### 1 triceps dips

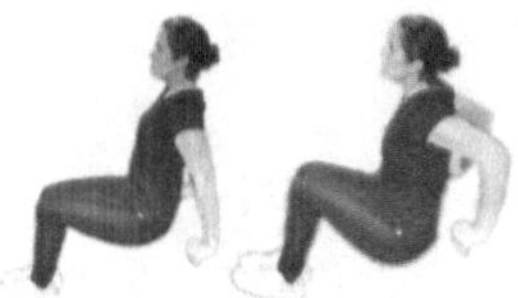

### 3 123 knee

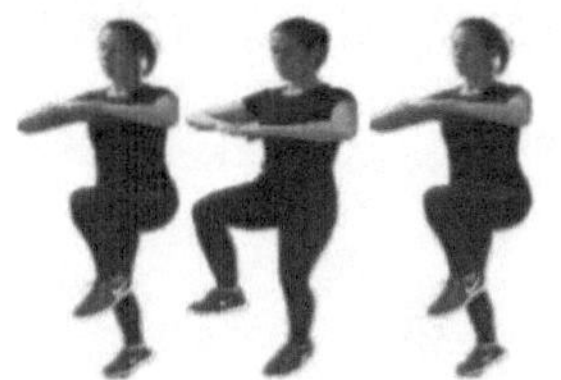

### 5 pushup jacks

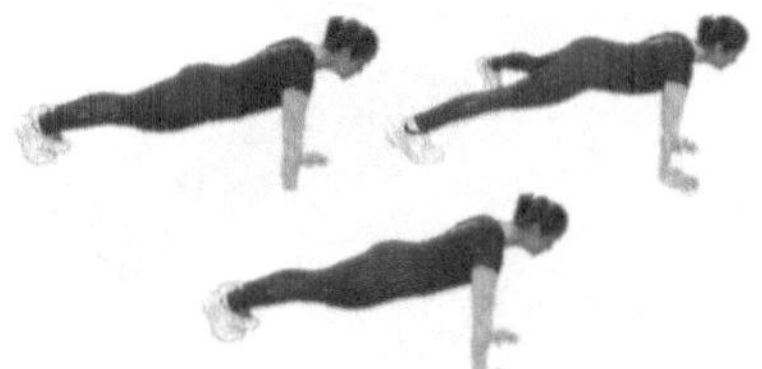

### 7 bicycles

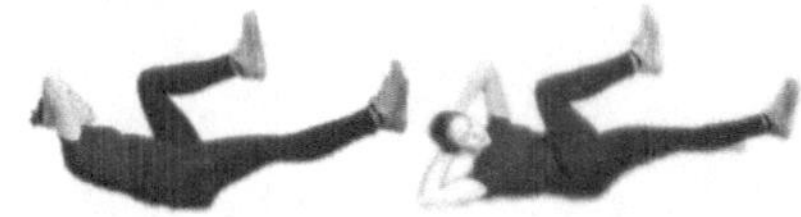

### 2 pioneer squats in and out

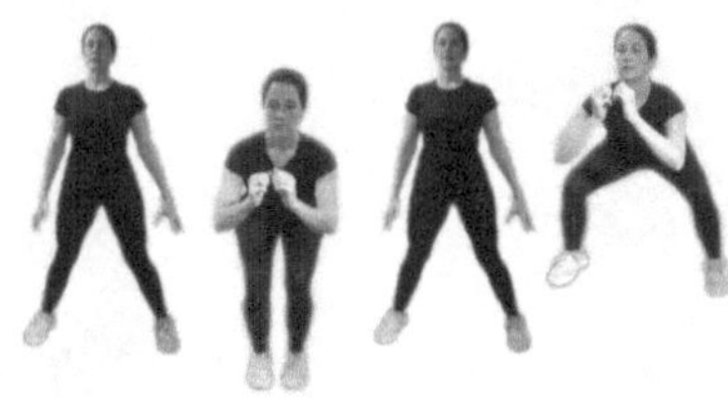

### 4 lateral shuffles

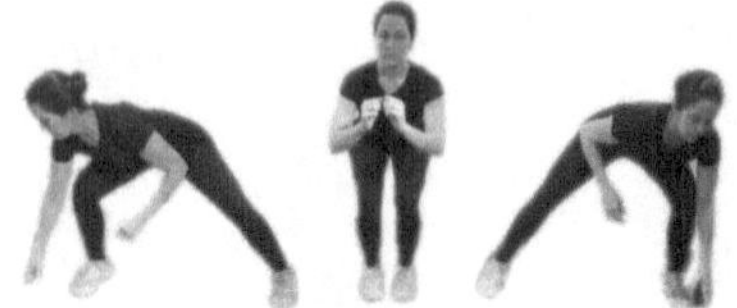

### 6 plank alternating leg lifts

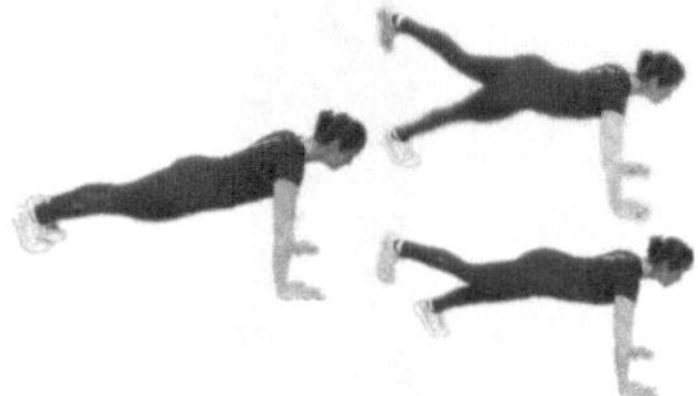

## Rest period between circuit rounds 2 min then begin circuits again.

## Cool down – 10 min- see page

Thursday Cardio & flexibility training
Week 2 pre-training

**2 x 5** min
warmup & cool down

**30** min
workout time

**40** min
total time

## Warm up -5 min

## Cardio - 30 min

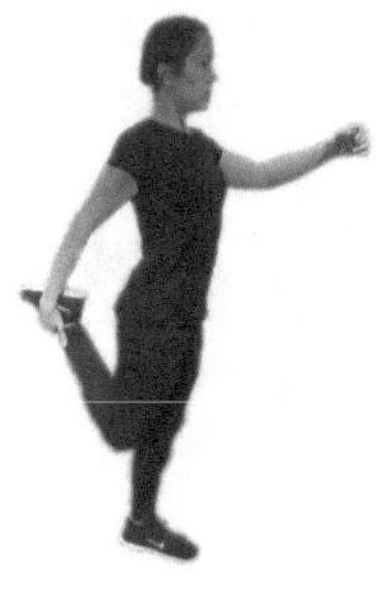

Quad stretch

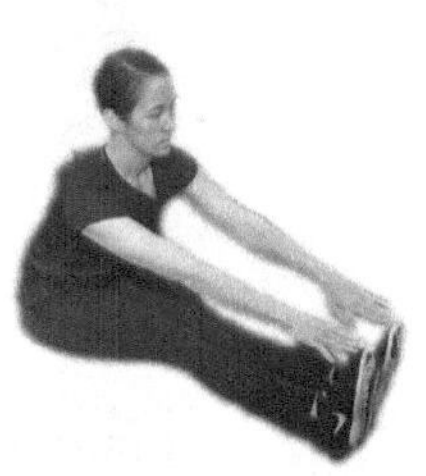

Hamstring stretch

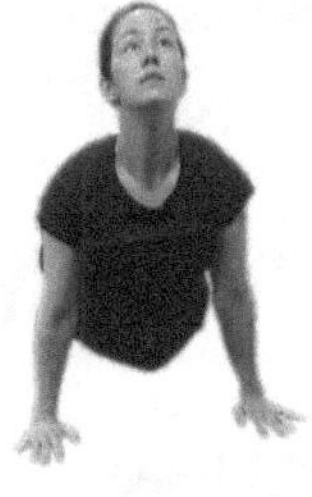

Abdominals

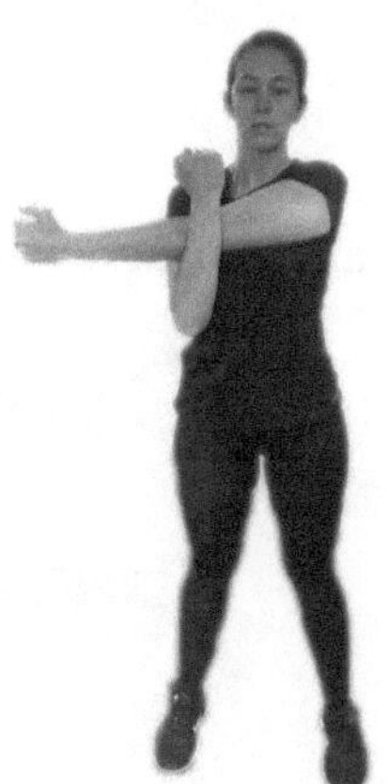

Upper back stretch

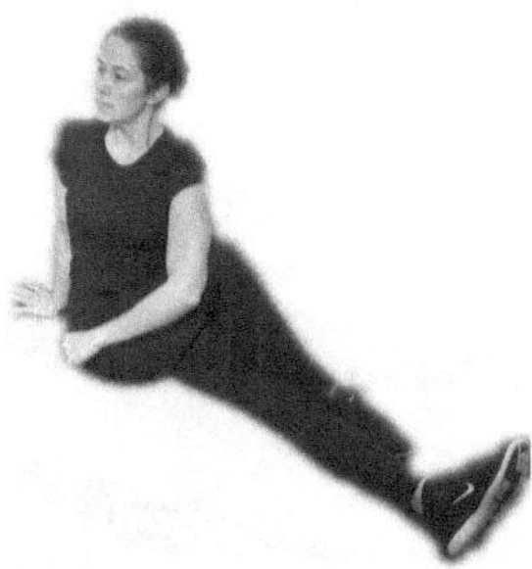

Rotational

## Make sure to follow stretches on page

## Cool down – 5 min- see page

Friday Pioneer Power Training
workout
Week 2

# 1 x 6 min
circuits

# 6 min
workout time

# 26 min
total time

## Warm up -10 min

## F.H.I.T Circuit - 7 min - Repeat 2 times

1 lateral lunge

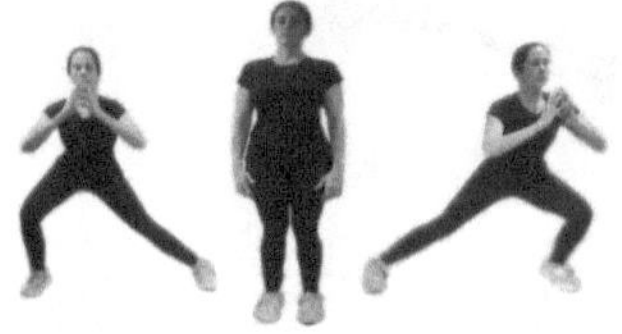

4 plank rotation

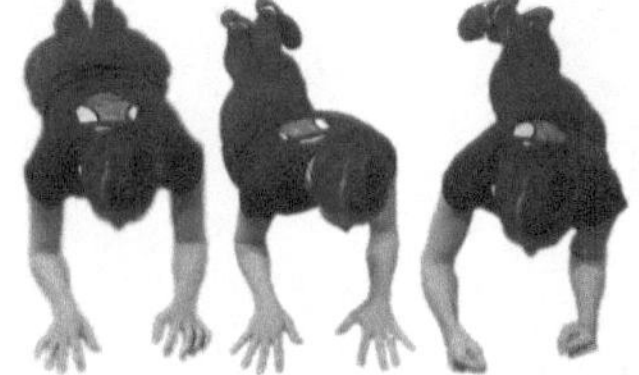

3 burpee

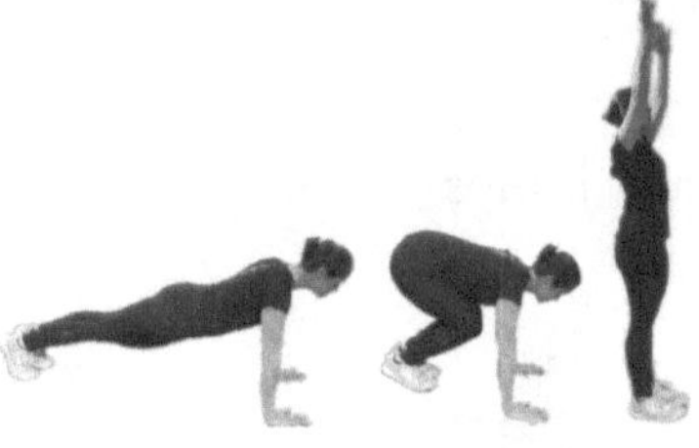

2 power jump

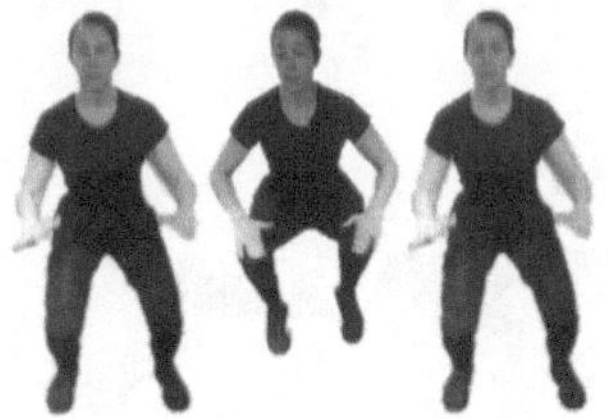

The 6minute clock is continuous. Continue to move through the circuit, performing the repetitions required.

## Cool down – 10 min- see page

Monday Functional High
Intensity Training workout
Week 3

**2 x 7** min
circuits

**14** min
workout time

**37** min
total time

## Warm up -10 min

## F.H.I.T Circuit - 7 min - Repeat 2 times

1 sumo squats

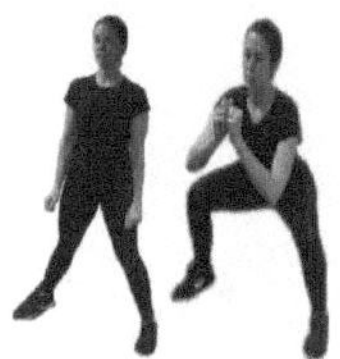

3 mountain climber

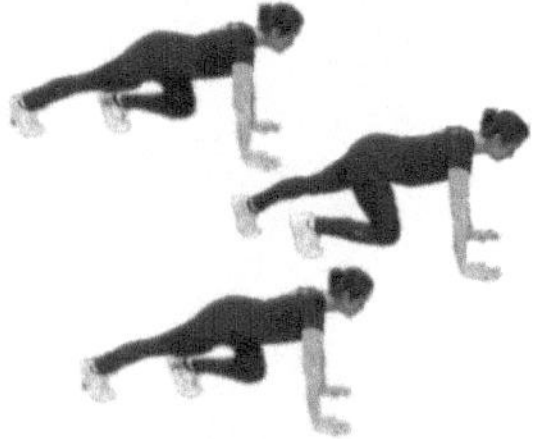

5 high knees

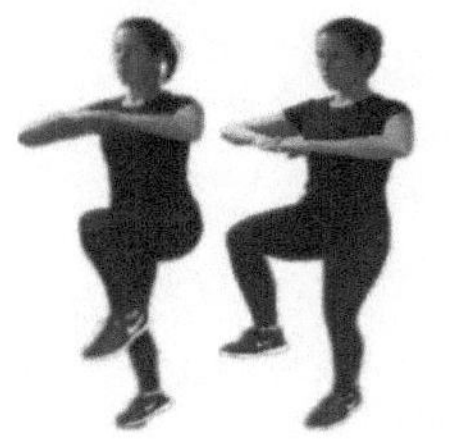

7 plank alternating leg lift

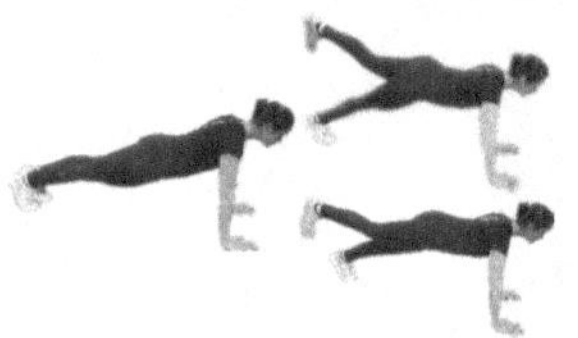

2 pushups

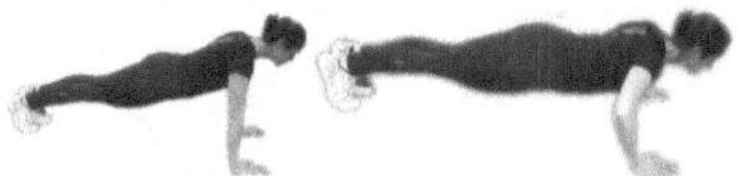

4 squat jumps

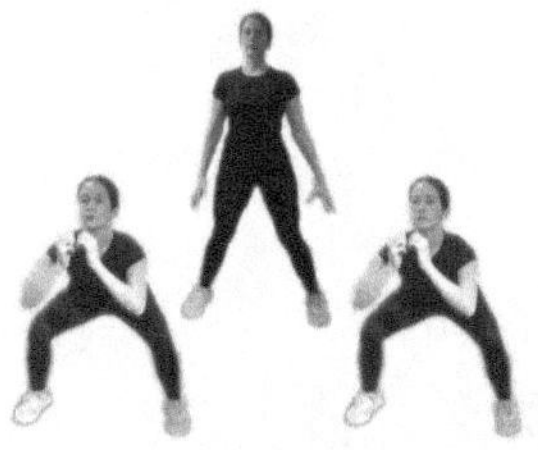

6 half burpees

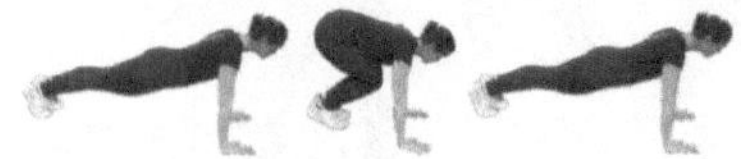

## Rest period between circuit rounds 2 min then begin circuits again.

## Cool down – 10 min- see page

Tuesday is recovery training

Week 3 pre-training

**2 x 5** min
warmup & cool down

**30** min
workout time

**40** min
total time

## Warm up -5 min

## Cardio - 30 min

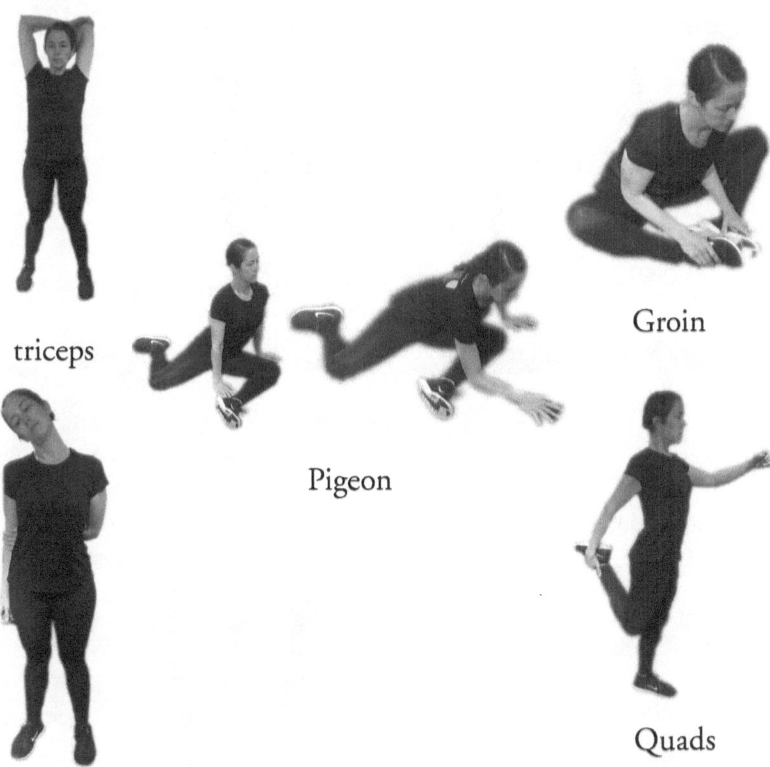

triceps

Pigeon

Groin

Quads

Neck & shoulder

## Make sure to follow stretches on page

## Cool down – 5 min- see page

Wednesday Functional High
Intensity Training workout
Week 3

**2 x 7** min
circuits

**14** min
workout time

**37** min
total time

## Warm up -10 min

## F.H.I.T Circuit - 7 min - Repeat 2 times

### 1 squat jumps

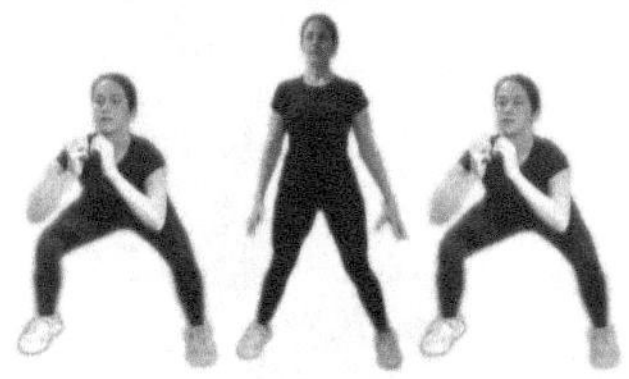

### 2 high knees

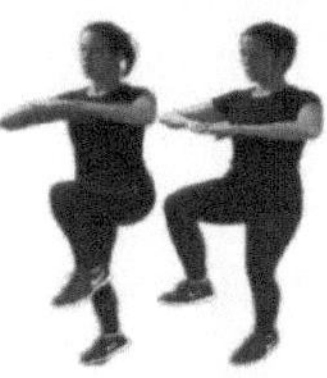

### 3 push ups

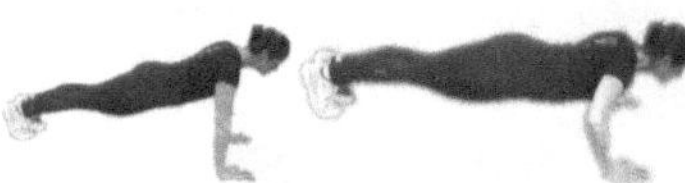

### 4 plank alternating knee

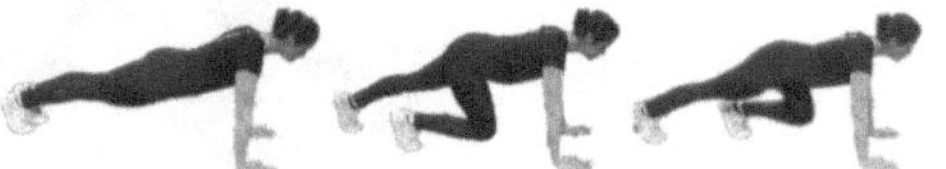

### 5 plank hip rotation

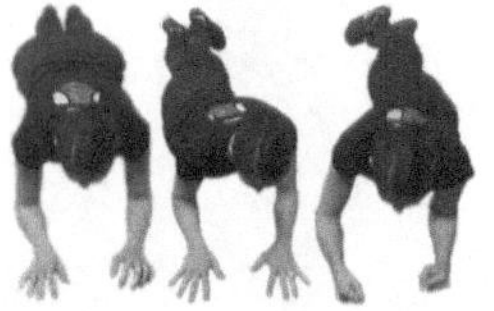

### 6 123 knee

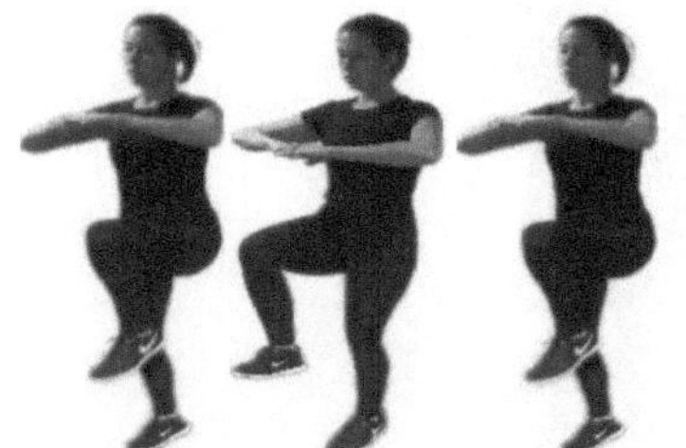

### 7 walking lunges

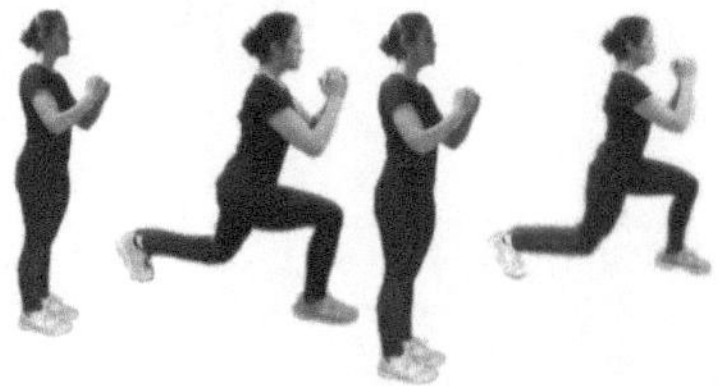

Rest period between circuit rounds 2 min then begin circuits again.

Cool down – 10 min- see page

Thursday Cardio & flexibility training

Week 3 pre-training

**2 x 5** min
warmup & cool down

**30** min
workout time

**40** min
total time

## Warm up -5 min

## Cardio - 30 min

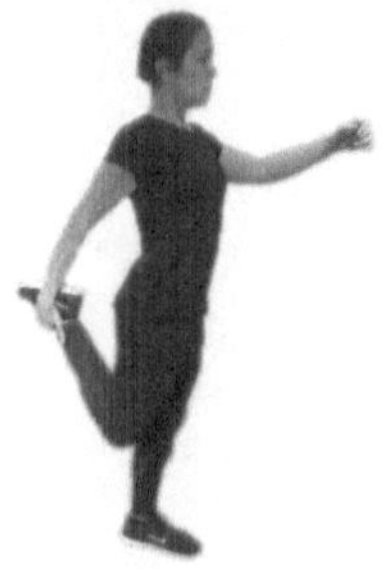

Quad stretch

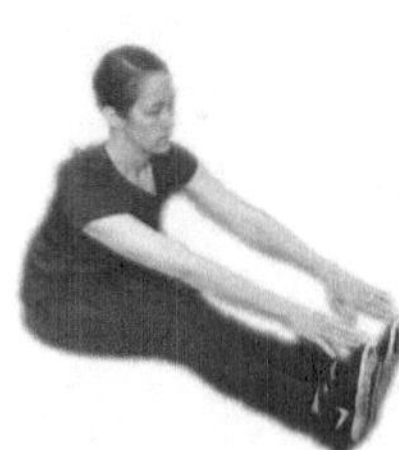

Hamstring stretch

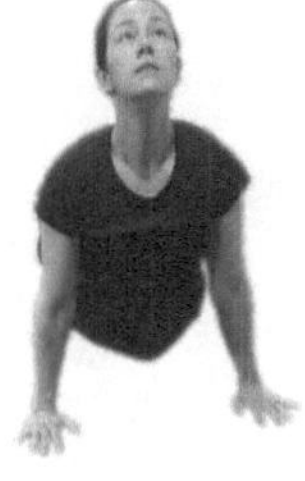

Abdominals

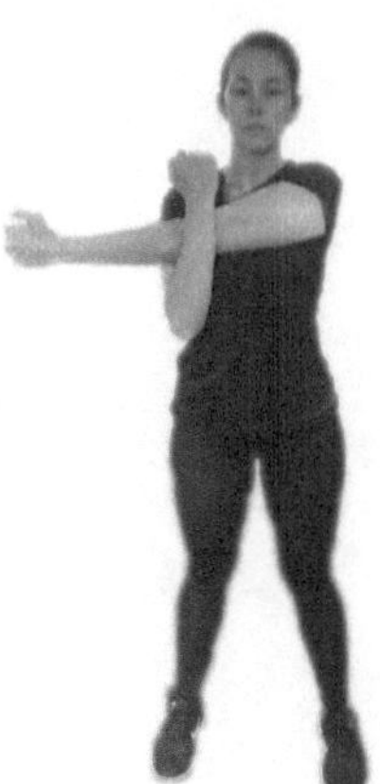

Upper back stretch

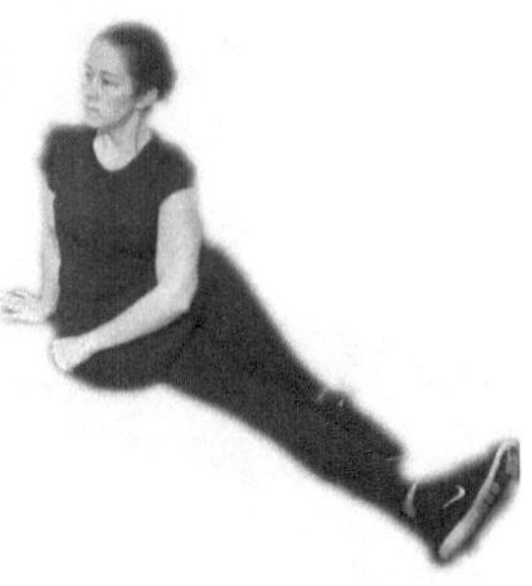

Rotational

Make sure to follow stretches on page

Cool down – 5 min- see page

Friday Pioneer Power Training workout

Week 3

**1 x 6** min
circuits

**6** min
workout time

**26** min
total time

## Warm up -10 min

## F.H.I.T Circuit - 7 min - Repeat 2 times

**1** glute bridges

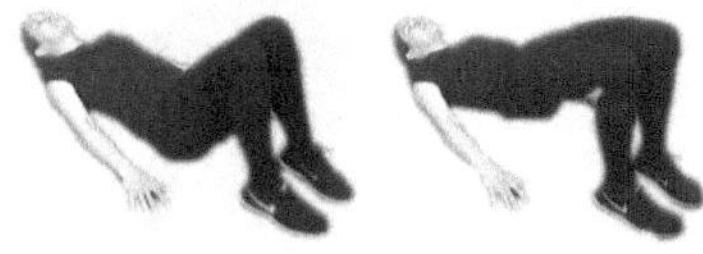

**3** power jump

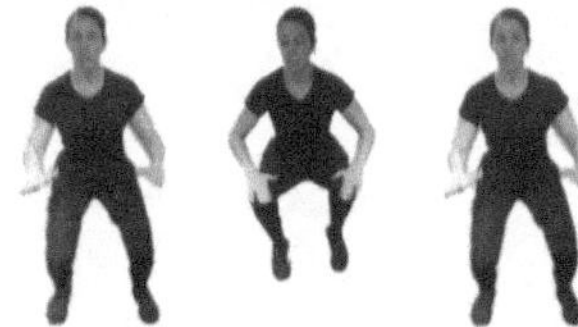

**2** half burpee

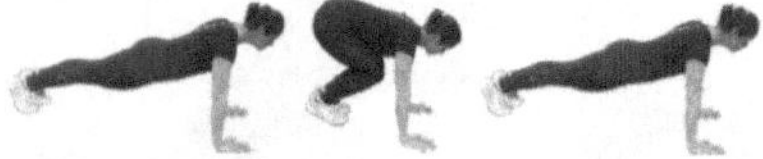

**4** bungees

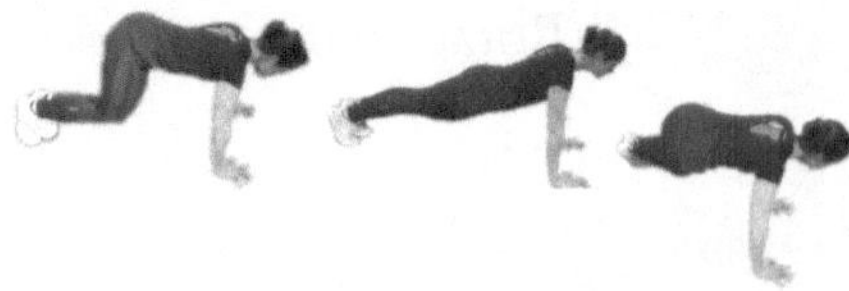

The 6minute clock is continuous. Continue to move through the circuit, performing the repetitions required.

Cool down – 10 min- see page

Monday Functional High
Intensity Training workout
Week 4

**2 x 7** min
circuits

**14** min
workout time

**37** min
total time

## Warm up -10 min

## F.H.I.T Circuit - 7 min - Repeat 2 times

### 1 split jumps

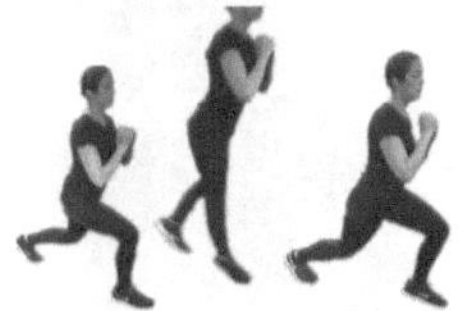

### 2 lateral shuffle

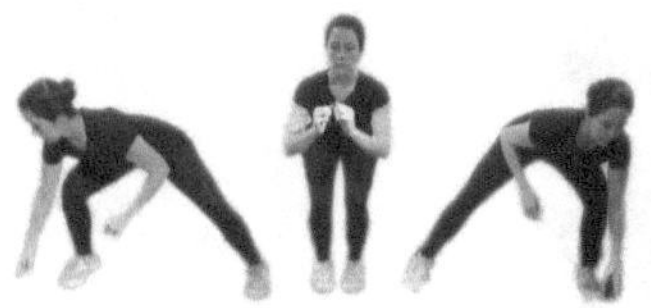

### 3 123 knee

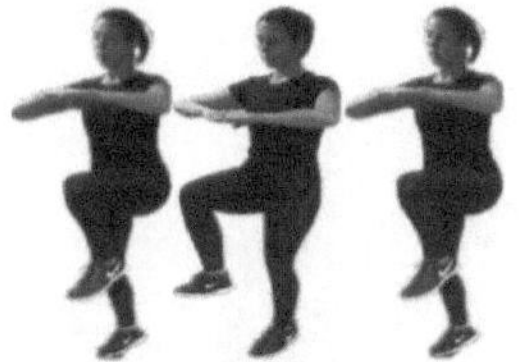

### 4 push up jack

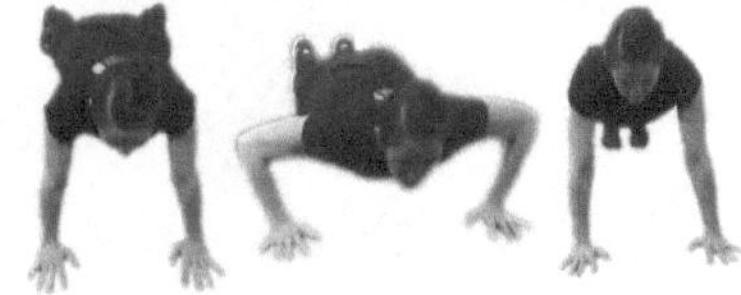

### 5 plank jacks

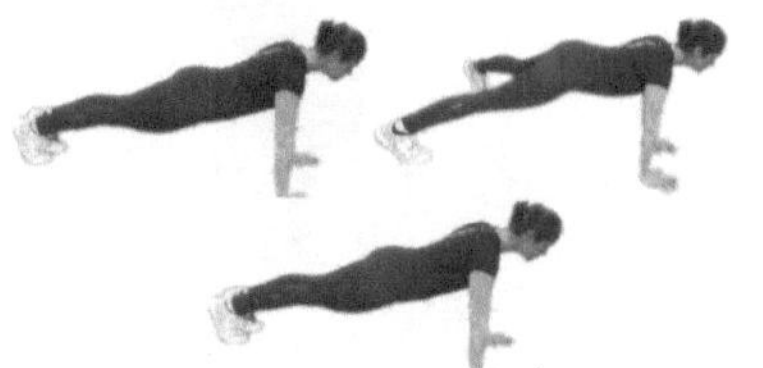

### 6 plank alternating leg lift

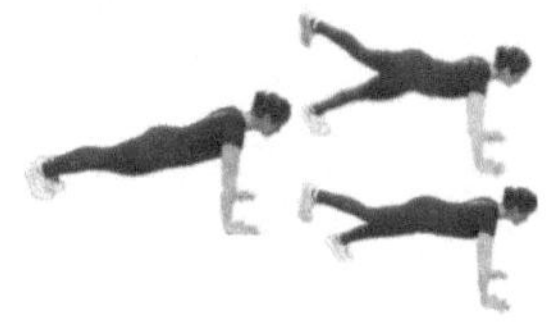

### 7 superman

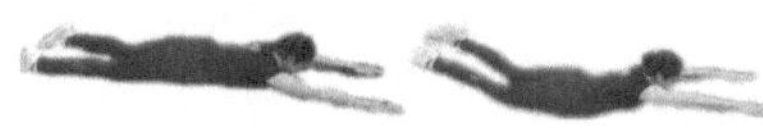

Rest period between circuit rounds 2 min then begin circuits again.

Cool down – 10 min- see page

Tuesday is recovery training

Week 4 pre-training

**2 x 5** min
warmup & cool down

**30** min
workout time

**40** min
total time

## Warm up -5 min

## Cardio - 30 min

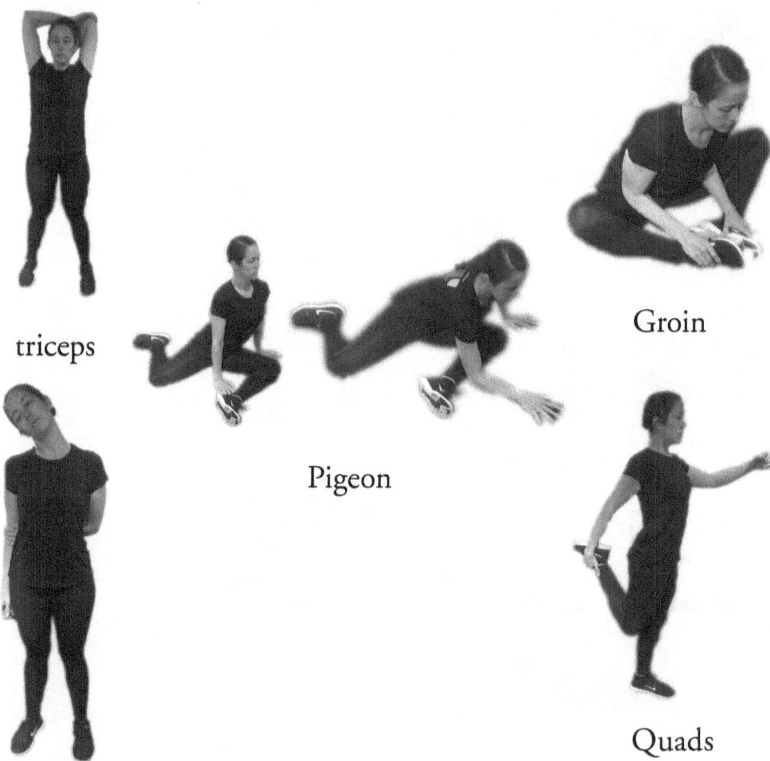

triceps

Pigeon

Groin

Neck & shoulder

Quads

## Make sure to follow stretches on page

## Cool down – 5 min- see page

Wednesday Functional High
Intensity Training workout
Week 4

**2 x 7** min
circuits

**14** min
workout time

**37** min
total time

## Warm up -10 min

## F.H.I.T Circuit - 7 min - Repeat 2 times

### 1 wide push ups

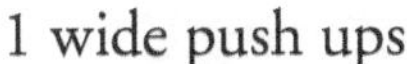

### 2 mountain climber

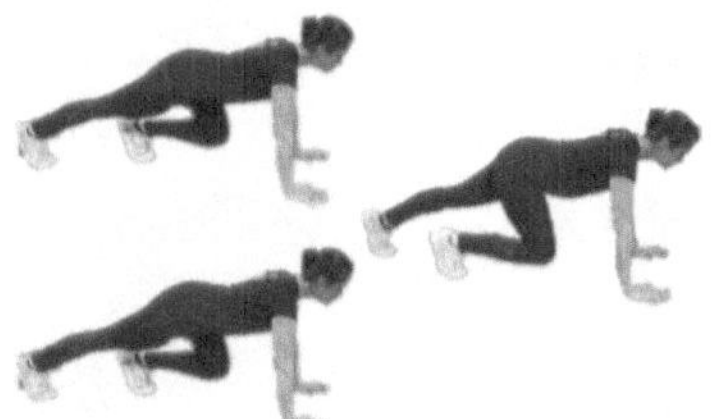

### 3 bungees

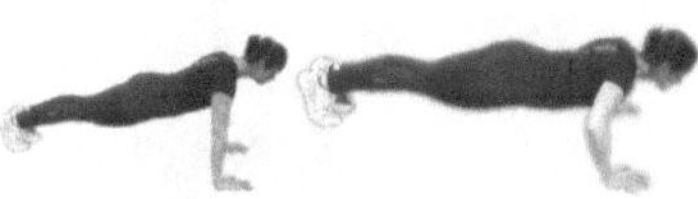

### 4 ladder climber

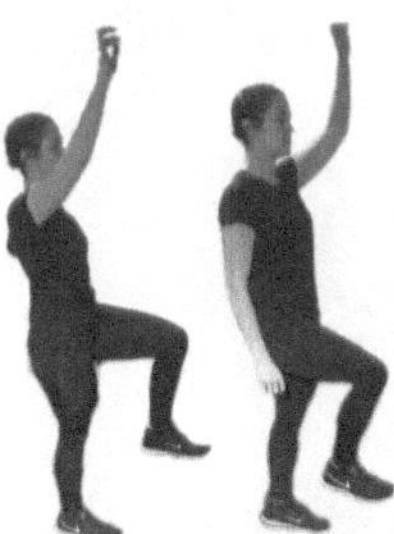

### 5 power jumps

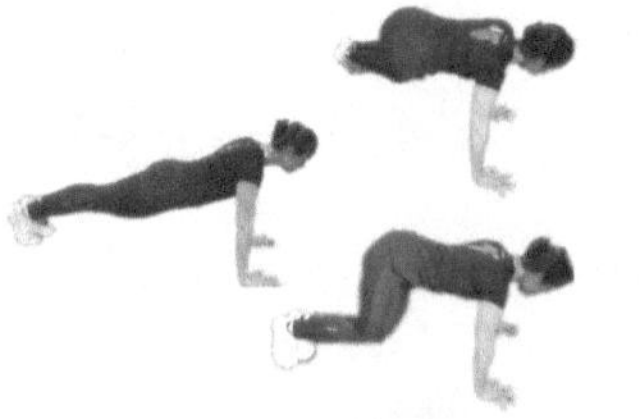

### 6 high knees

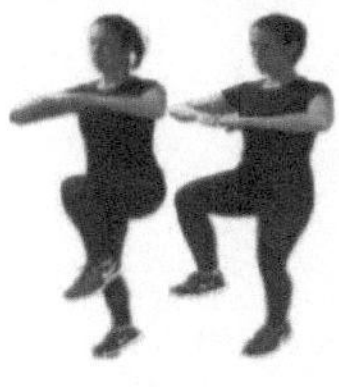

### 7 bicycles

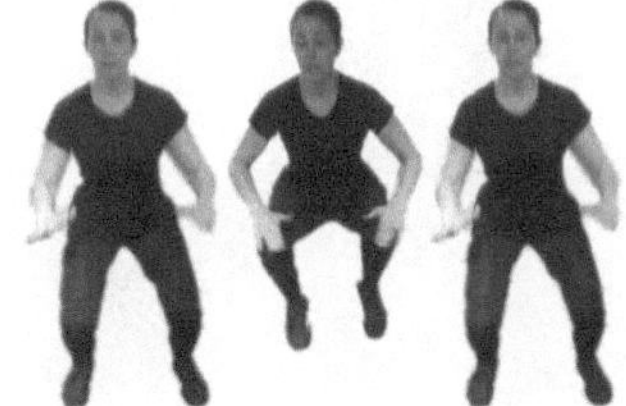

Rest period between circuit rounds 2 min then begin circuits again.

Cool down – 10 min- see page

Thursday Cardio & flexibility training
Week 4 pre-training

**2 x 5** min
warmup & cool down

**30**min
workout time

**40**min
total time

## Warm up -5 min

## Cardio - 30 min

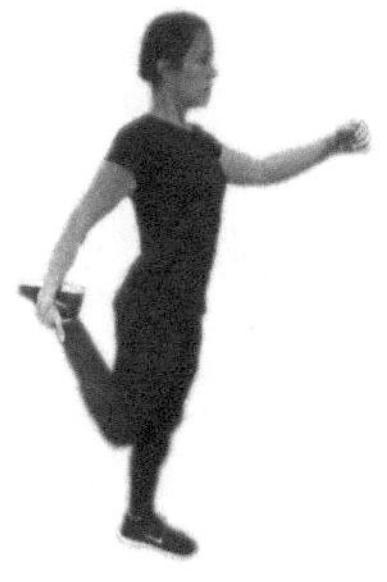

Quad stretch

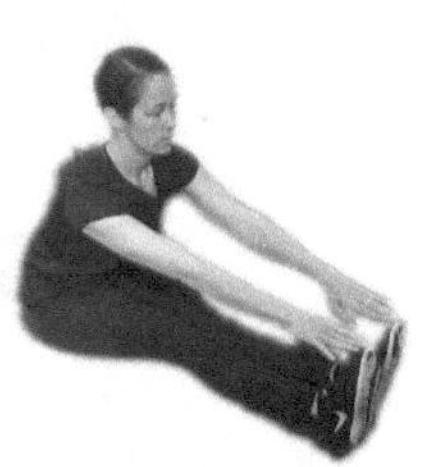

Hamstring stretch

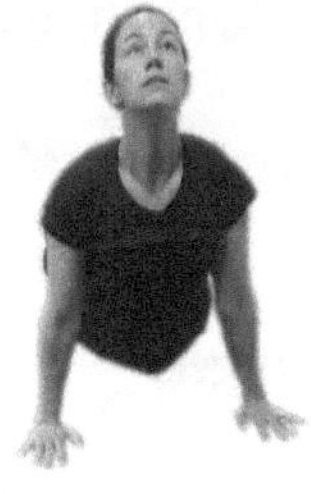

Abdominals

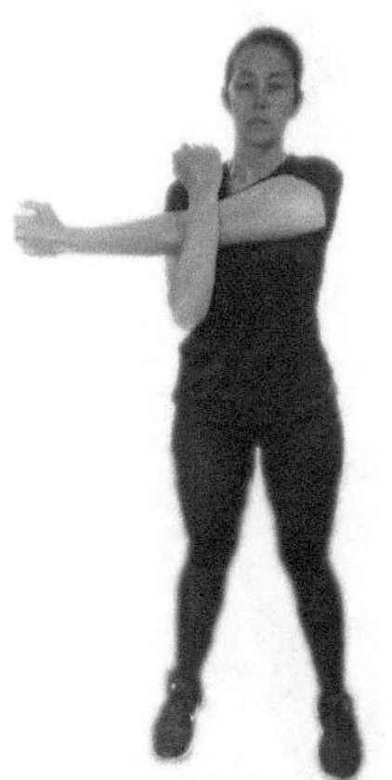

Upper back stretch

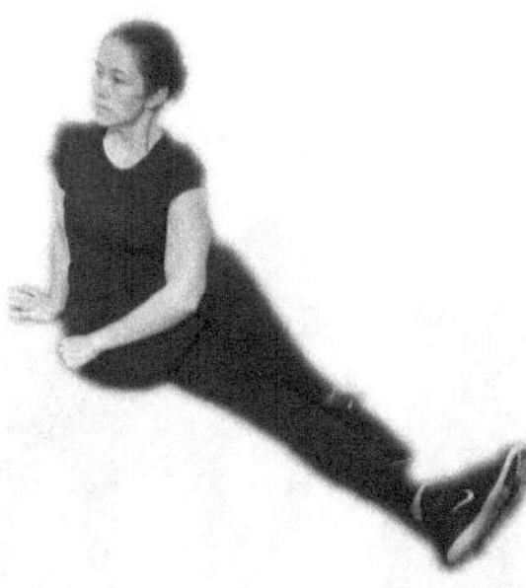

Rotational

## Make sure to follow stretches on page

## Cool down – 5 min- see page

Friday Pioneer Power Training workout
Week 4

**1 x 6**min
circuits

**6**min
workout time

**26**min
total time

## Warm up -10 min

## F.H.I.T Circuit - 7 min - Repeat 2 times

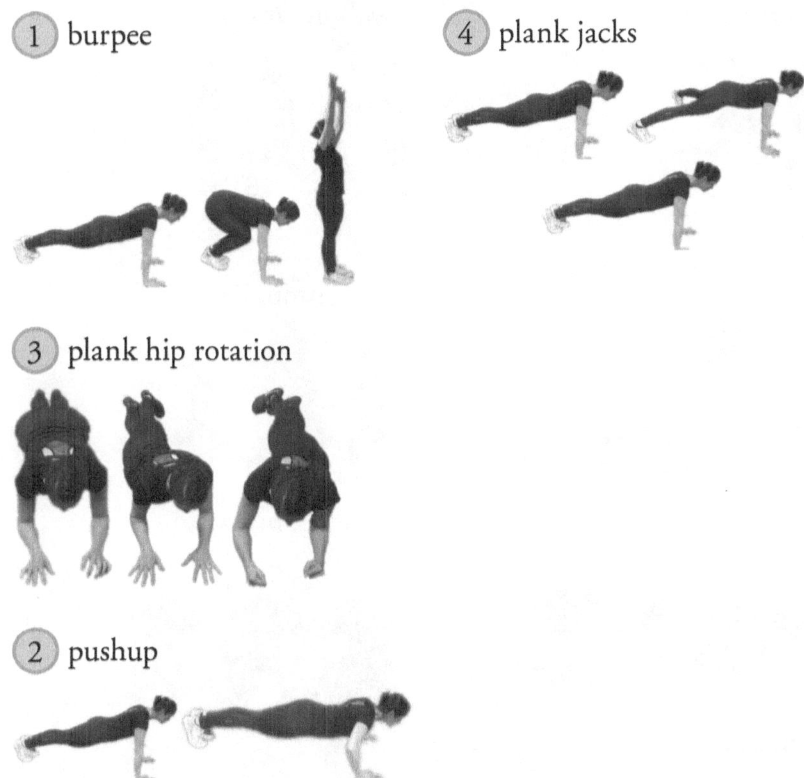

( 1 ) burpee

( 4 ) plank jacks

( 3 ) plank hip rotation

( 2 ) pushup

The 6minute clock is continuous. Continue to move through the circuit, performing the repetitions required.

Cool down – 10 min- see page

Monday Functional High
Intensity Training workout
Week 5

**2 x 7** min
circuits

**14** min
workout time

**37** min
total time

## Warm up -10 min

## F.H.I.T Circuit - 7 min - Repeat 2 times

### 1 sumo squats

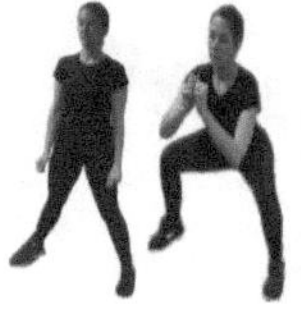

### 2 walking lunge

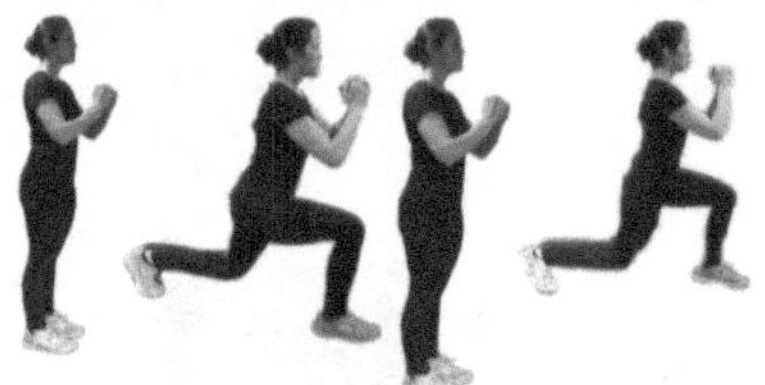

### 3 squat jumps

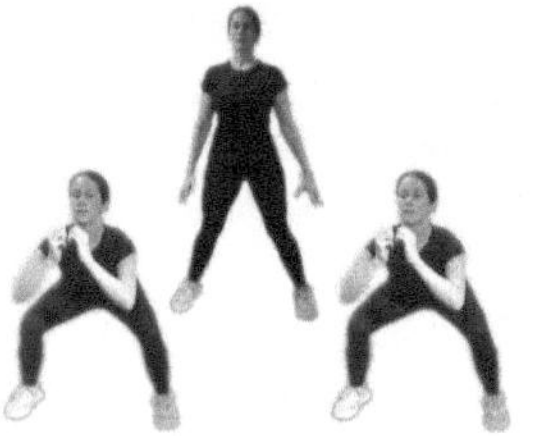

### 4 split jumps

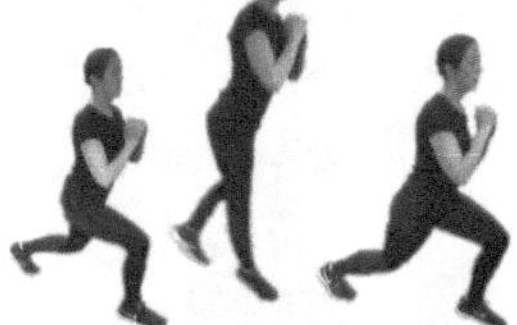

### 5 glute bridge

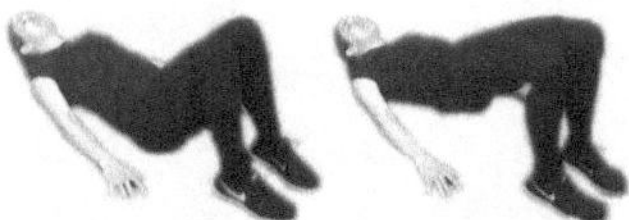

### 6 power jumps

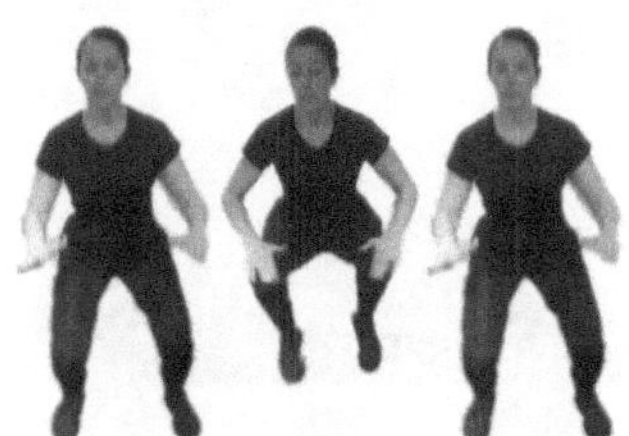

### 7 robot pushups

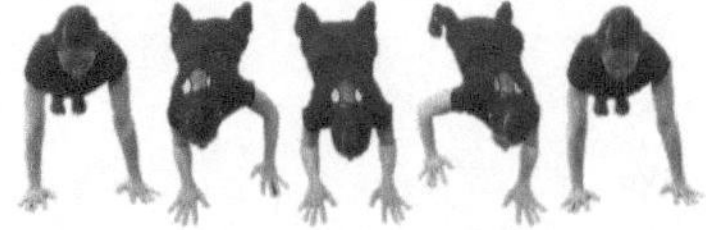

## Rest period between circuit rounds 2 min then begin circuits again.

## Cool down – 10 min- see page

Tuesday is recovery training

Week 5 pre-training

**2 x 5** min
warmup & cool down

**30**min
workout time

**40**min
total time

## Warm up -5 min

## Cardio - 30 min

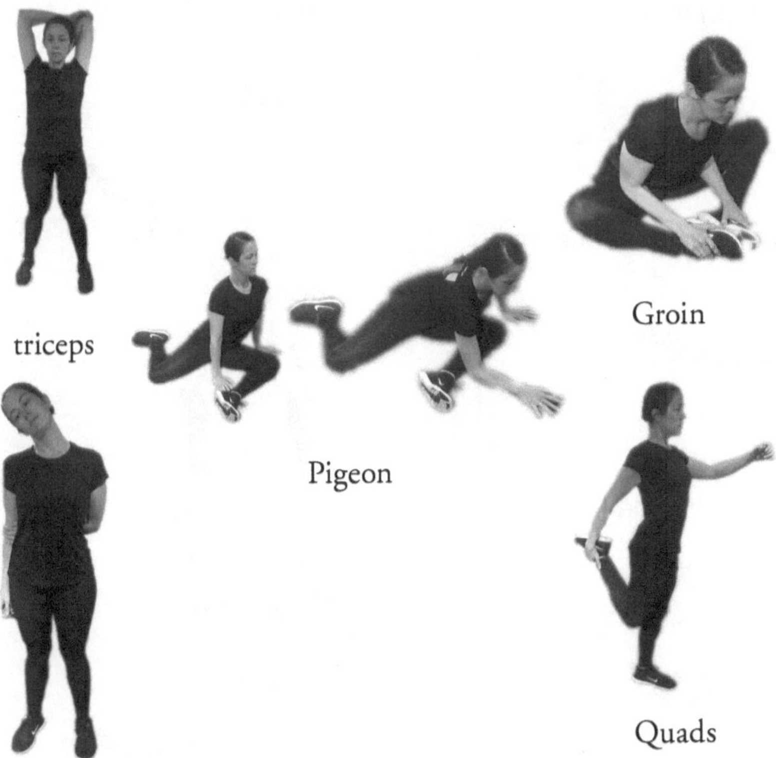


## Make sure to follow stretches on page

## Cool down – 5 min- see page

Wednesday Functional High
Intensity Training workout
Week 5

**2 x 7** min
circuits

**14** min
workout time

**37** min
total time

## Warm up -10 min

## F.H.I.T Circuit - 7 min - Repeat 2 times

1 split jumps

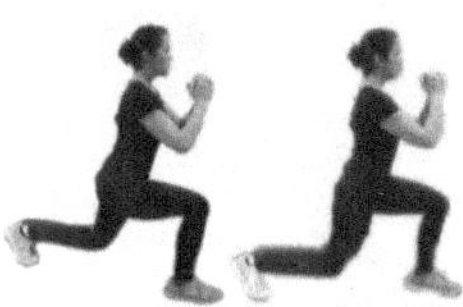

2 v ups

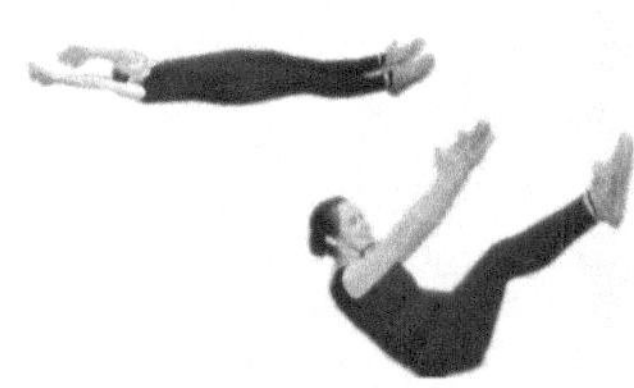

3 plank alternating leg lift

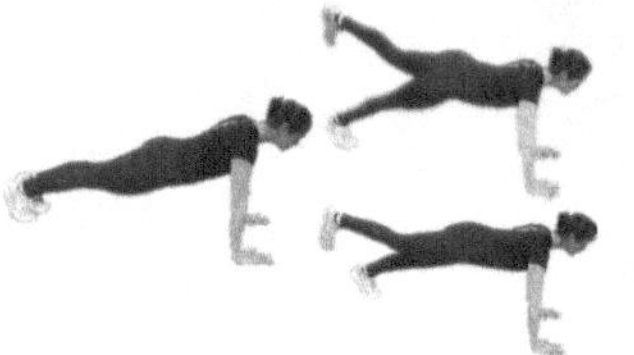

4 back lunge

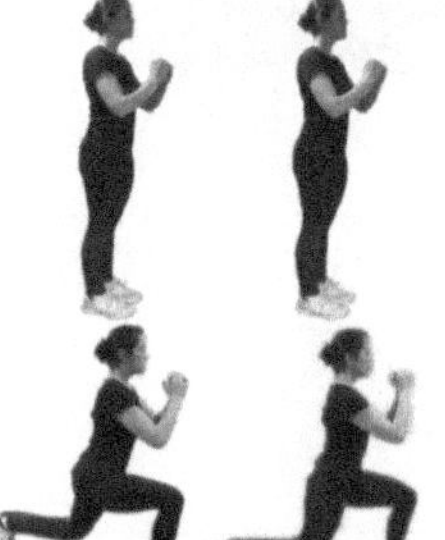

5 mountain climbers

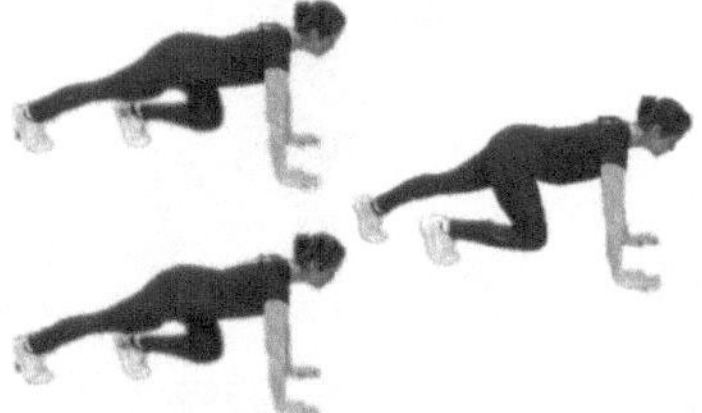

6 bungees

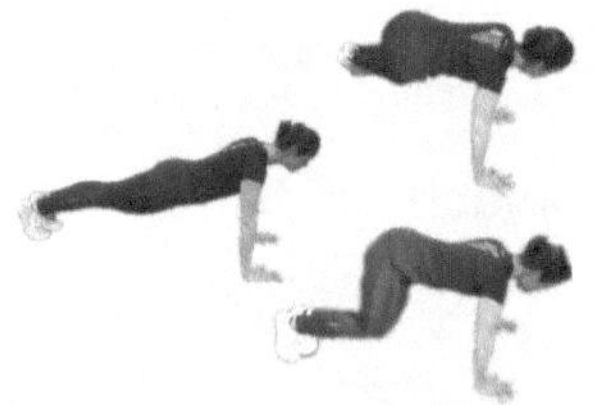

7 plank alt knees

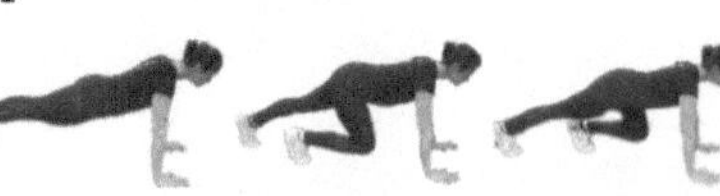

Rest period between circuit rounds 2 min then begin circuits again.

Cool down – 10 min- see page

Thursday Cardio & flexibility training
Week 5 pre-training

**2 x 5** min
warmup & cool down

**30** min
workout time

**40** min
total time

## Warm up -5 min

## Cardio - 30 min

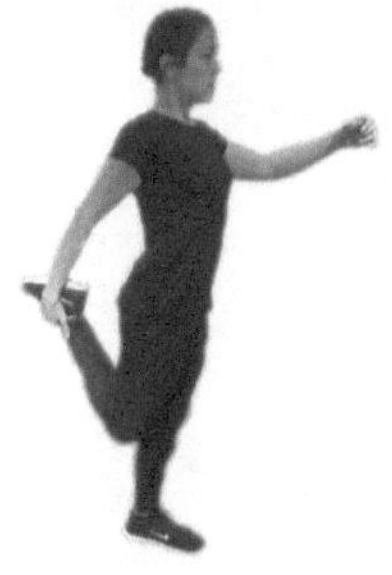

Quad stretch

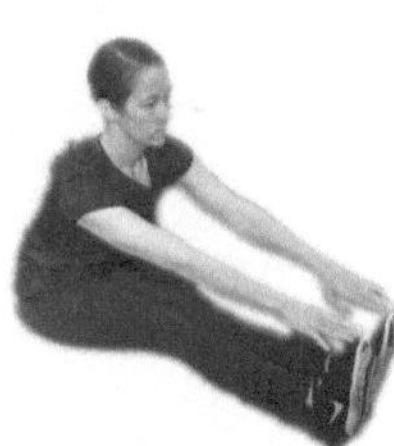

Hamstring stretch

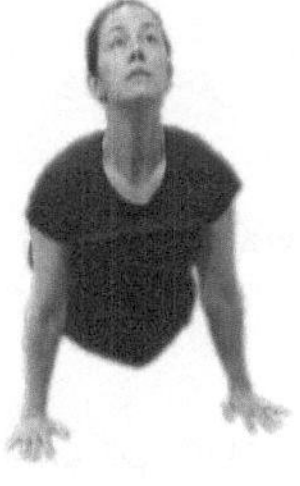

Abdominals

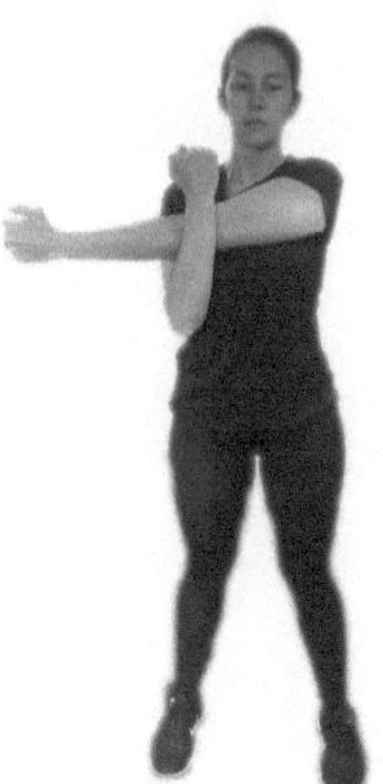

Upper back stretch

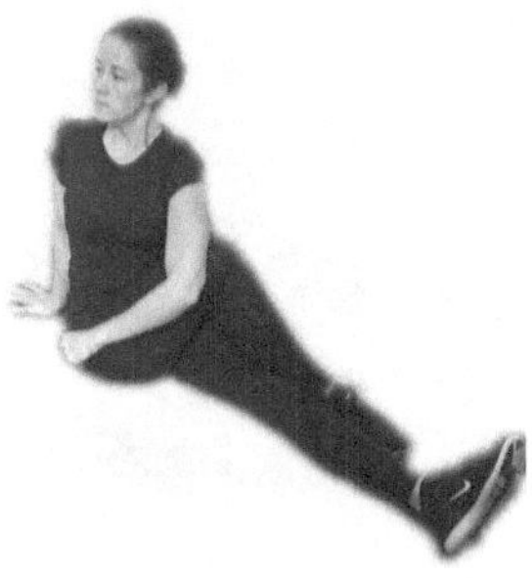

Rotational

## Make sure to follow stretches on page

## Cool down – 5 min- see page

Friday Pioneer Power Training workout
Week 5

**1 x 6** min
circuits

**6** min
workout time

**26** min
total time

## Warm up -10 min

## F.H.I.T Circuit - 7 min - Repeat 2 times

**1** pushups

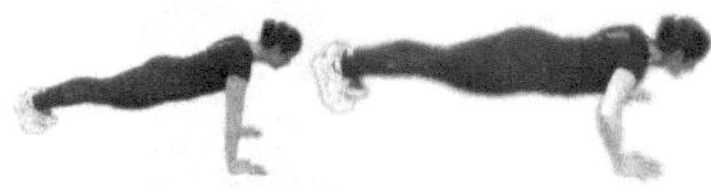

**3** triceps dips

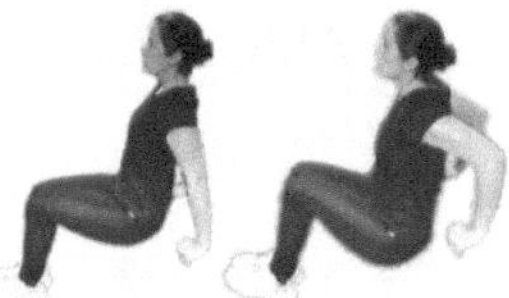

**2** plank jacks

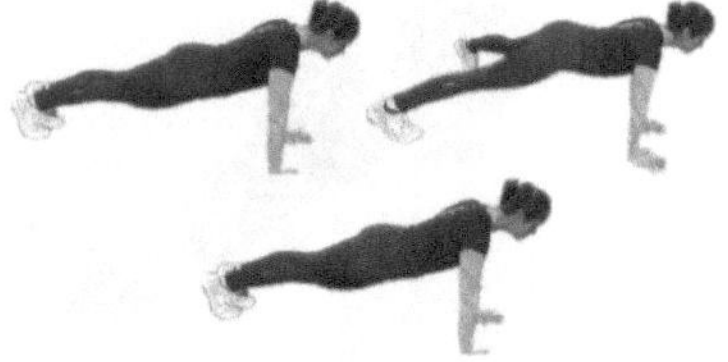

**4** superman

The 6minute clock is continuous. Continue to move through the circuit, performing the repetitions required.

Cool down – 10 min- see page

Monday Functional High Intensity Training workout
Week 6

**2 x 7** min
circuits

**14** min
workout time

**37** min
total time

## Warm up -10 min

## F.H.I.T Circuit - 7 min - Repeat 2 times

### 1 ski bumps

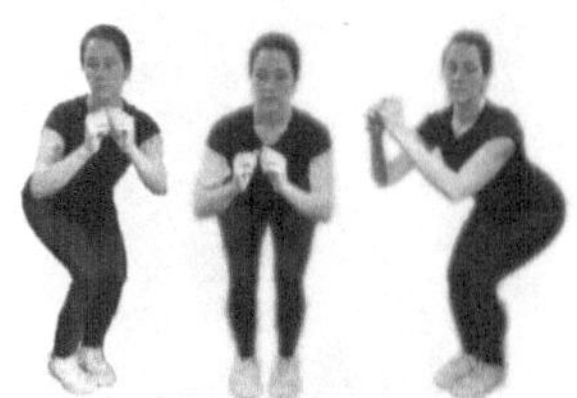

### 3 123 knee

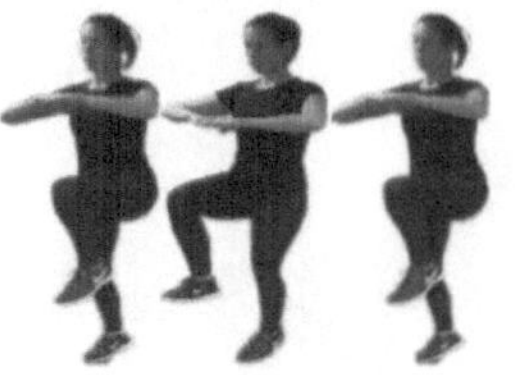

### 5 back lunges

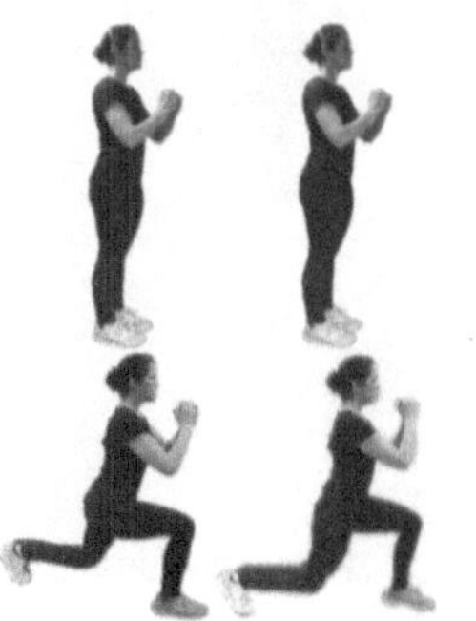

### 7 robot pushups

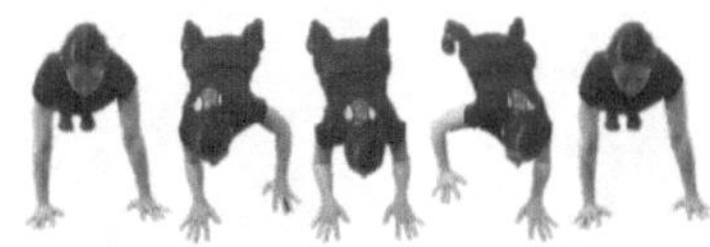

### 2 front and back hops

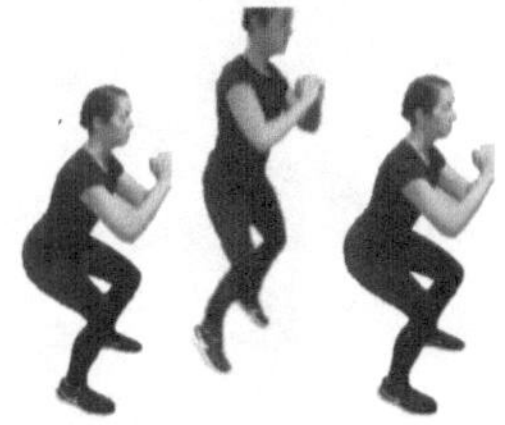

### 4 glute bridge

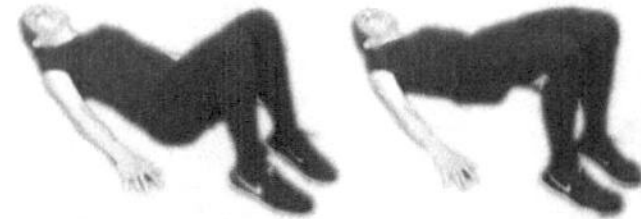

### 6 split jumps

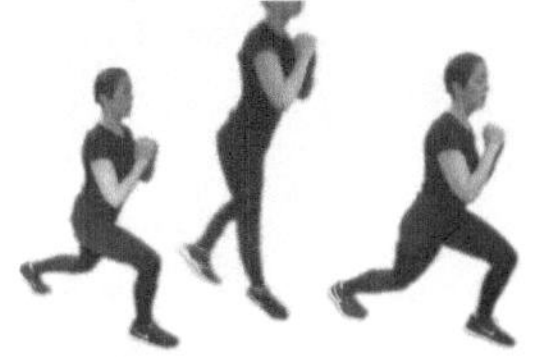

## Rest period between circuit rounds 2 min then begin circuits again.

## Cool down – 10 min- see page

Tuesday is recovery training

Week 6 pre-training

**2 x 5** min
warmup & cool down

**30** min
workout time

**40** min
total time

## Warm up -5 min

## Cardio - 30 min

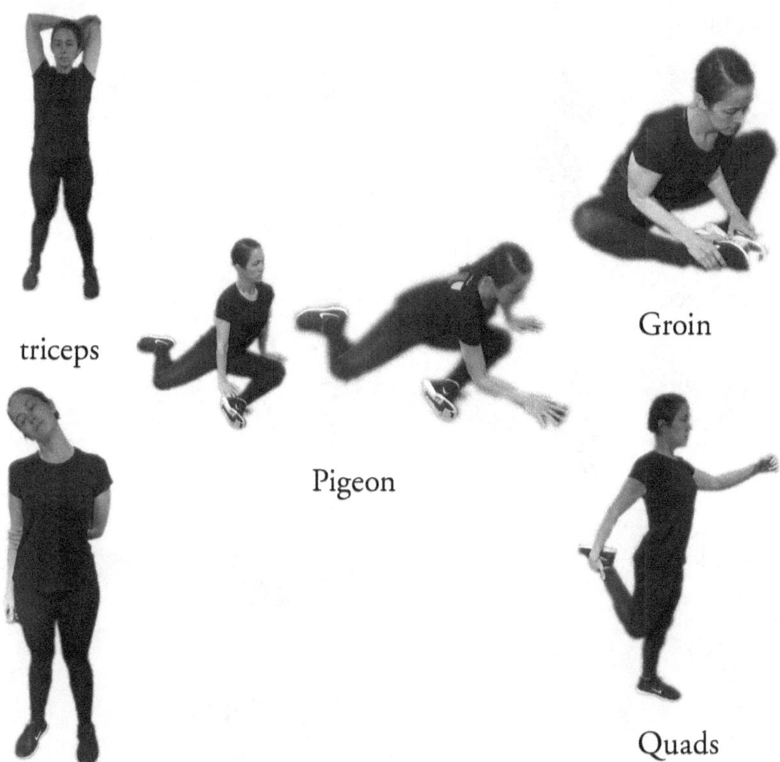

triceps

Pigeon

Groin

Neck & shoulder

Quads

## Make sure to follow stretches on page

## Cool down – 5 min- see page

Wednesday Functional High
Intensity Training workout
Week 6

**2 x 7** min
circuits

**14** min
workout time

**37** min
total time

## Warm up -10 min

## F.H.I.T Circuit - 7 min - Repeat 2 times

1 2 push up and move

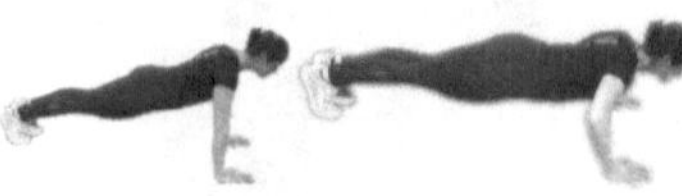

3 plank alternating leg lift

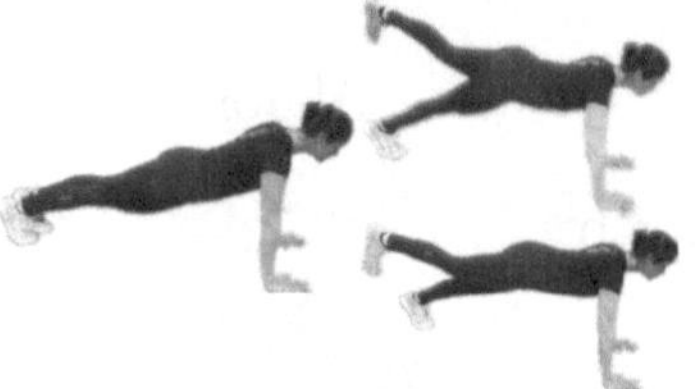

5 half burpees

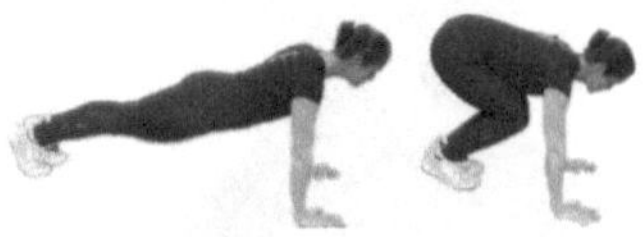

7 bungees

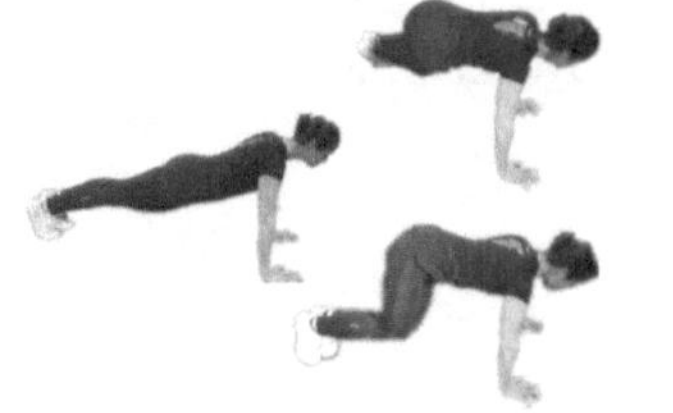

2 triceps dips

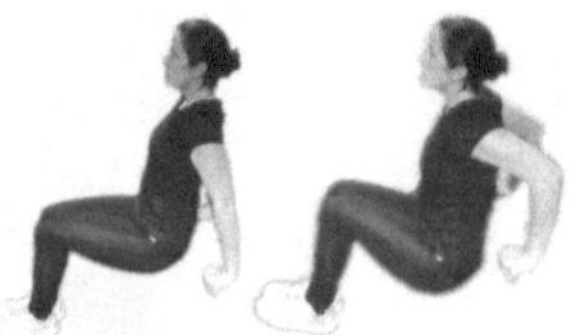

4 plank alternating arm lifts

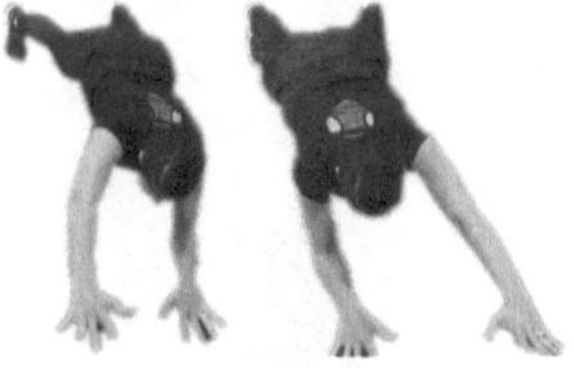

6 mountain climbers

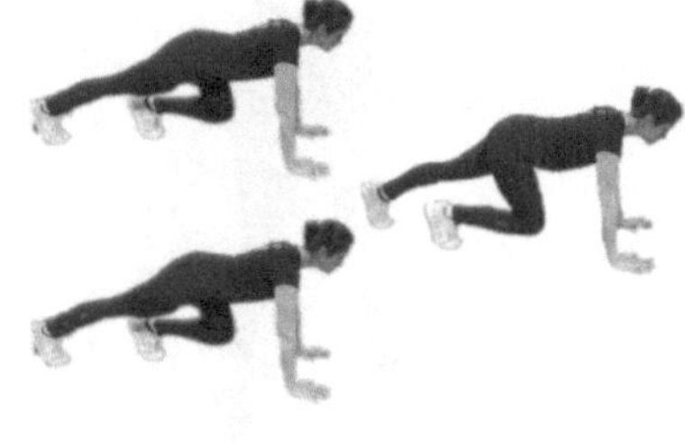

Rest period between circuit rounds 2 min then begin circuits again.

Cool down – 10 min- see page

Thursday Cardio & flexibility training

Week 6 pre-training

**2 x 5** min
warmup & cool down

**30** min
workout time

**40** min
total time

## Warm up -5 min

## Cardio - 30 min

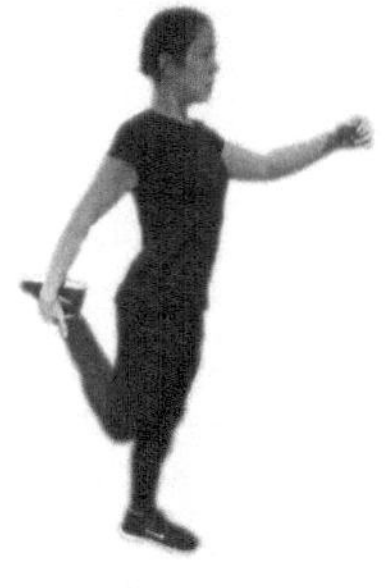

Quad stretch

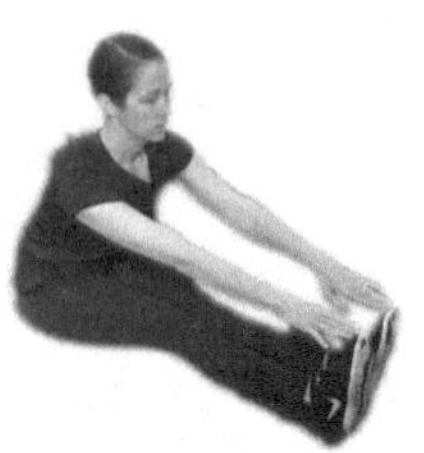

Hamstring stretch

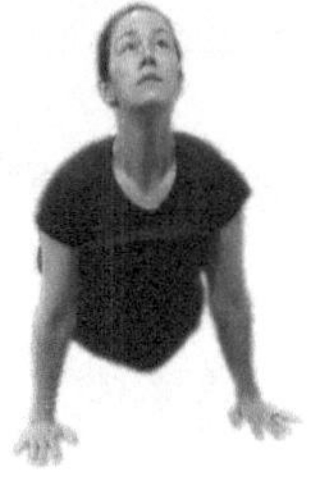

Abdominals

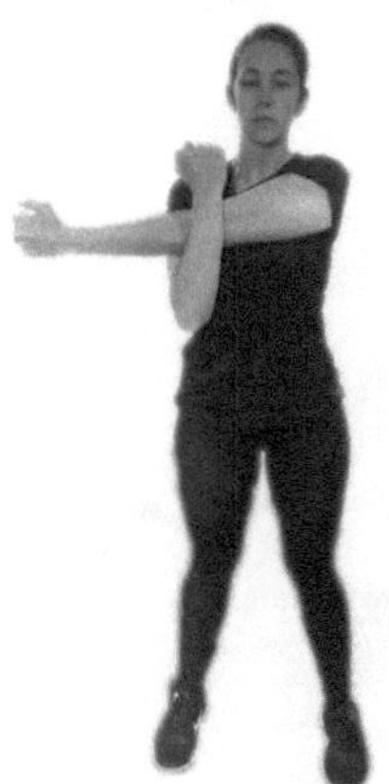

Upper back stretch

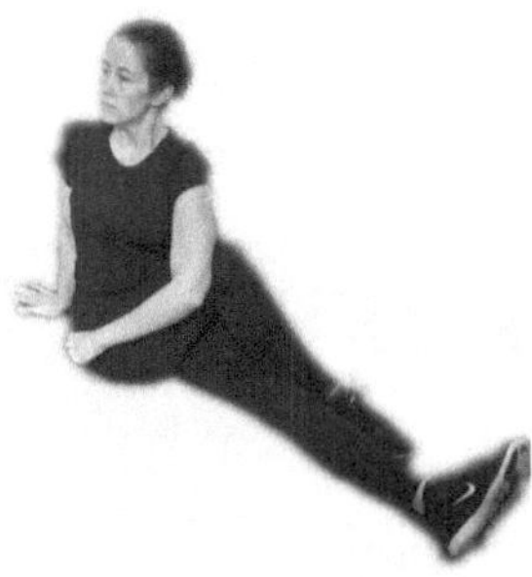

Rotational

## Make sure to follow stretches on page

## Cool down – 5 min- see page

Friday Pioneer Power Training workout
Week 6

**1 x 6** min
circuits

**6** min
workout time

**26** min
total time

## Warm up -10 min

## F.H.I.T Circuit - 7 min - Repeat 2 times

① power jumps

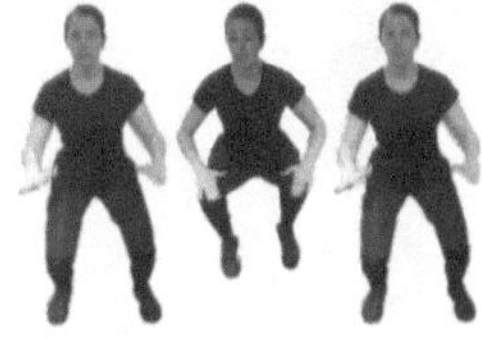

③ lateral towel jumps

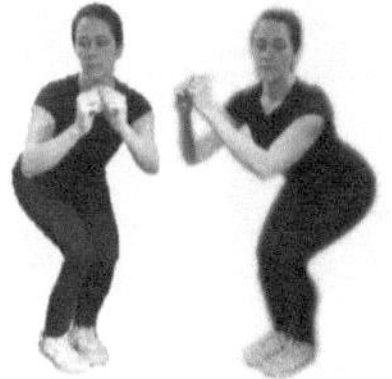

② burpee

④ plank alternating knees

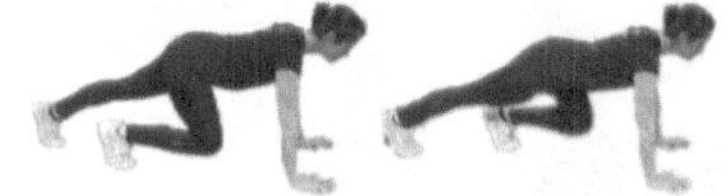

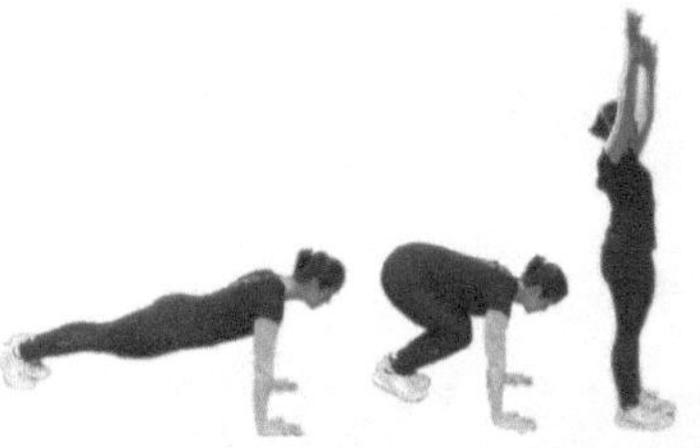

The 6minute clock is continuous. Continue to move through the circuit, performing the repetitions required.

## Cool down – 10 min- see page

Monday Functional High
Intensity Training workout
Week 7

**2 x 7** min
circuits

**14** min
workout time

**37** min
total time

## Warm up -10 min

## F.H.I.T Circuit - 7 min - Repeat 2 times

1 front and back hops

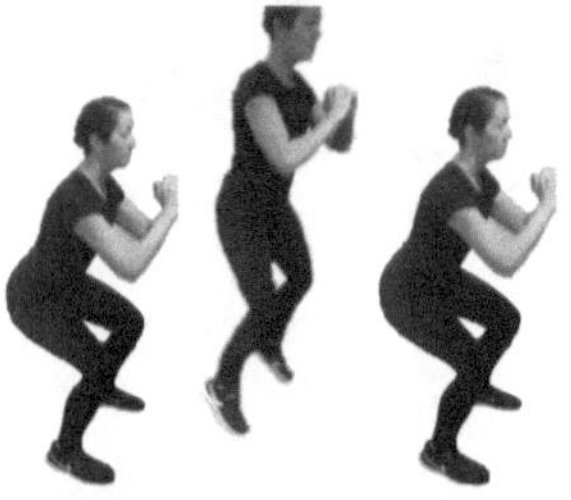

3 squat with side kick

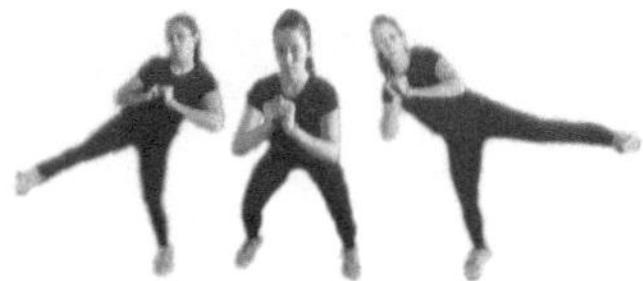

5 bungee

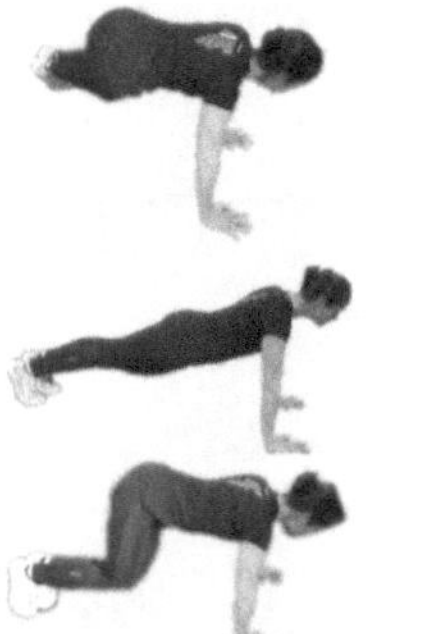

7 high knee

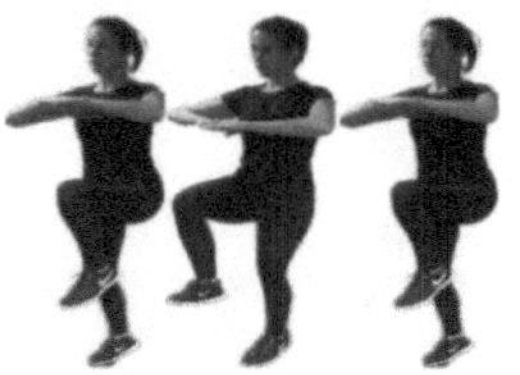

2 lateral lunges

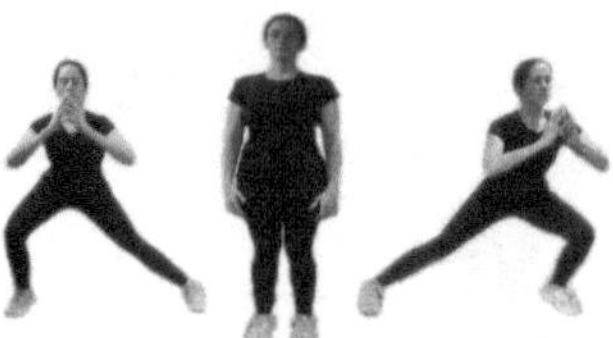

4 plank jacks

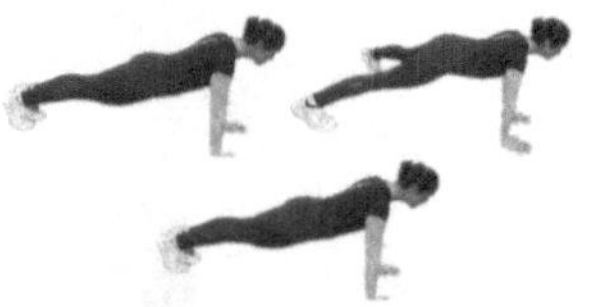

6 glute bridges

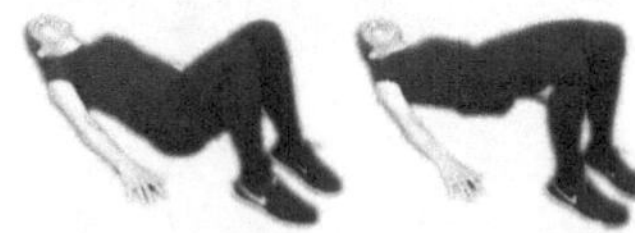

Rest period between circuit rounds 2 min then begin circuits again.

Cool down – 10 min- see page

Tuesday is recovery training

Week 7 pre-training

**2 x 5** min
warmup & cool down

**30** min
workout time

**40** min
total time

## Warm up -5 min

## Cardio - 30 min

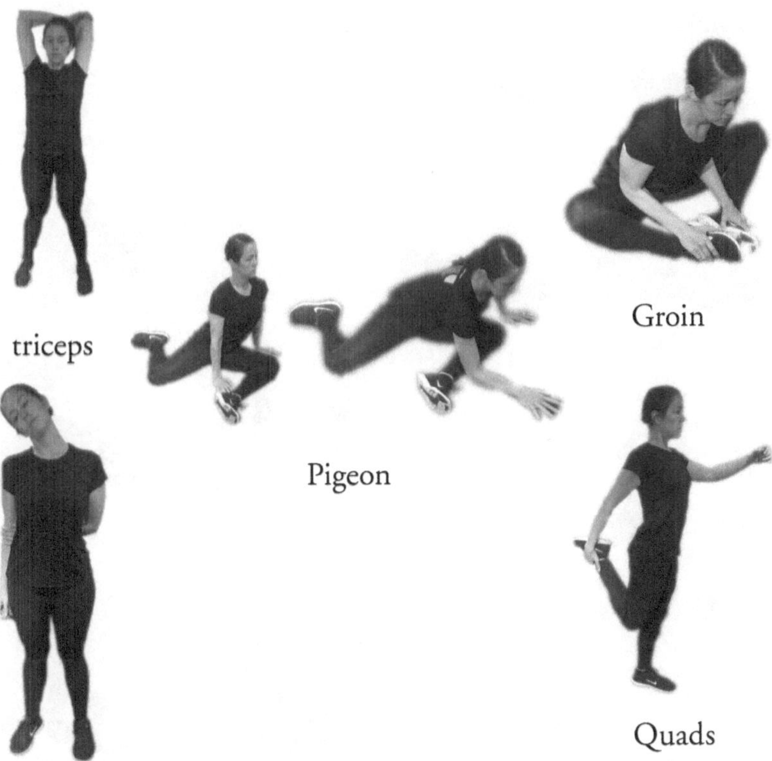


Make sure to follow stretches on page

Cool down – 5 min- see page

Wednesday Functional High
Intensity Training workout
Week 7

**2 x 7** min
circuits

**14** min
workout time

**37** min
total time

## Warm up -10 min

## F.H.I.T Circuit - 7 min - Repeat 2 times

### 1 incline pushup

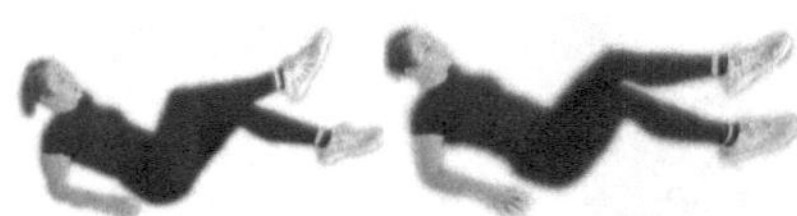

### 2 v ups

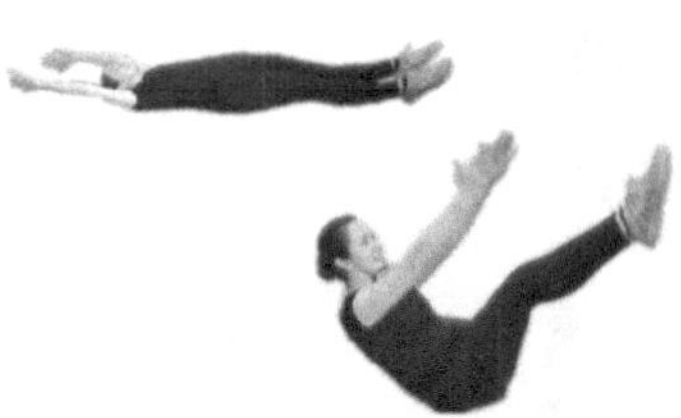

### 3 flutter kicks

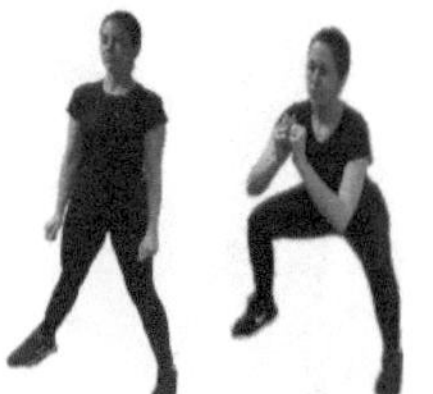

### 4 mountain climber

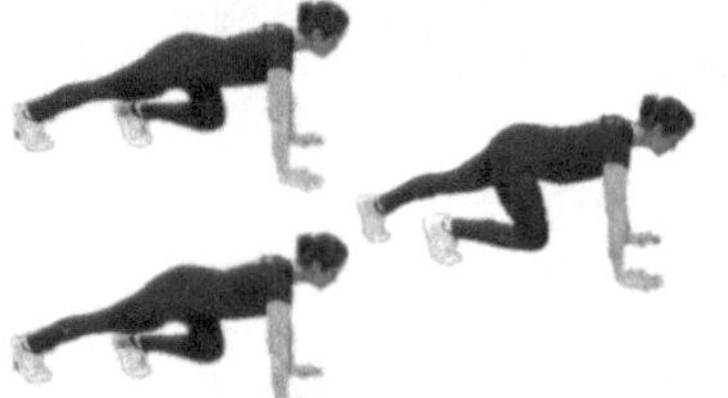

### 5 sumo squats

### 6 ab bicycles

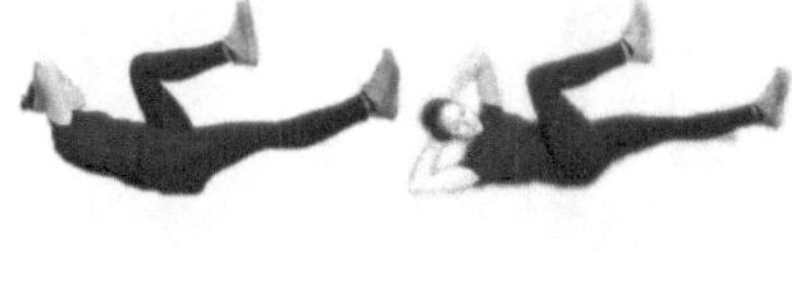

### 7 sit through

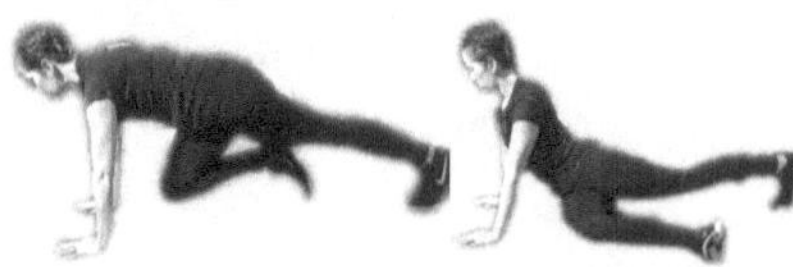

Rest period between circuit rounds 2 min then begin circuits again.

Cool down – 10 min- see page

Thursday Cardio & flexibility training
Week 7 pre-training

**2 x 5** min
warmup & cool down

**30** min
workout time

**40** min
total time

## Warm up -5 min

## Cardio - 30 min

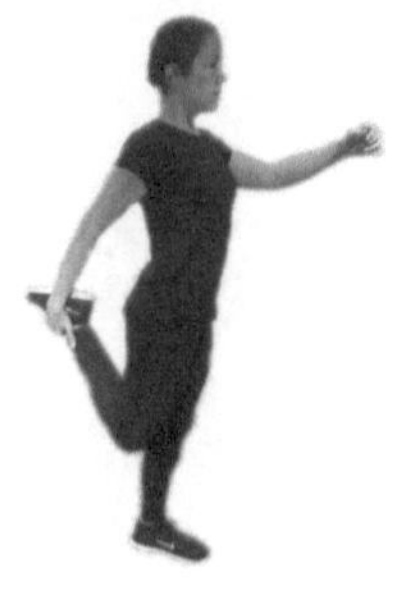

Quad stretch

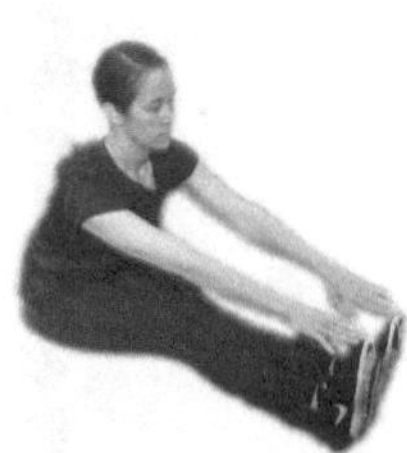

Hamstring stretch

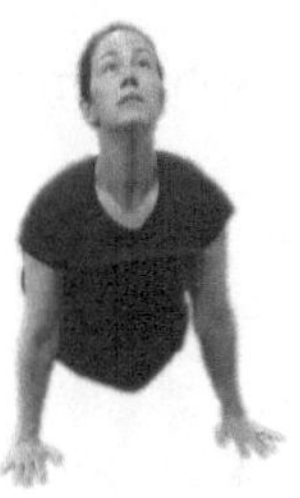

Abdominals

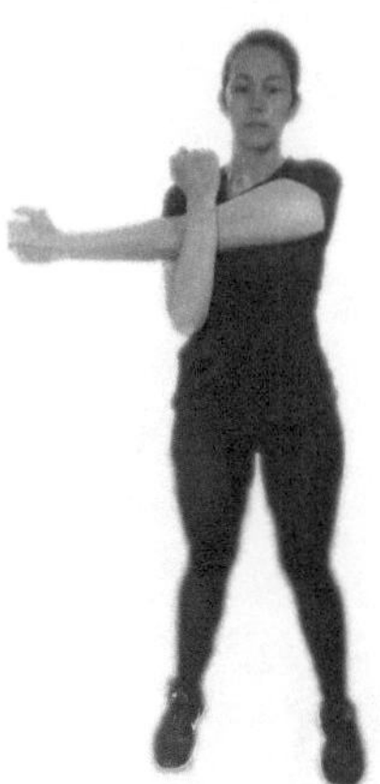

Upper back stretch

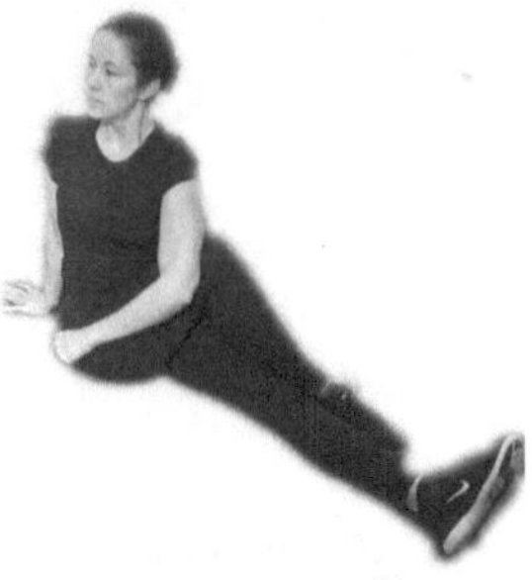

Rotational

## Make sure to follow stretches on page

## Cool down – 5 min- see page

Friday Pioneer Power Training
workout
Week 7

**1 x 6** min
circuits

**6** min
workout time

**26** min
total time

## Warm up -10 min

## F.H.I.T Circuit - 7 min - Repeat 2 times

**1** split jumps

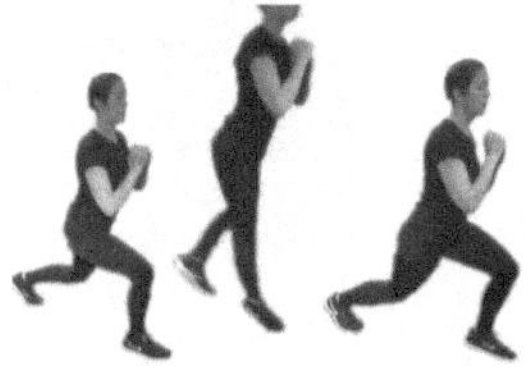

**3** plank alternating leg lift

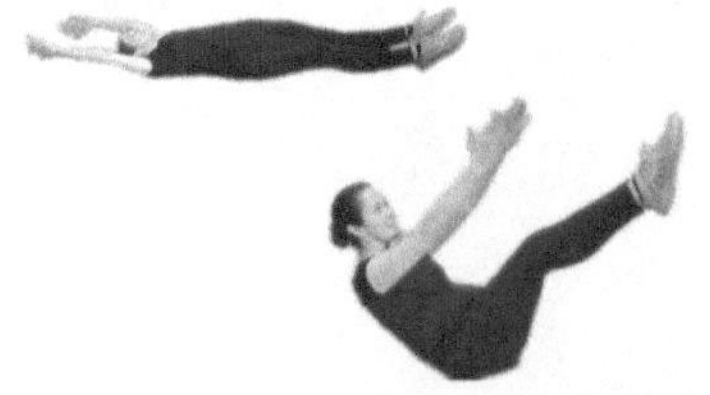

**2** v ups

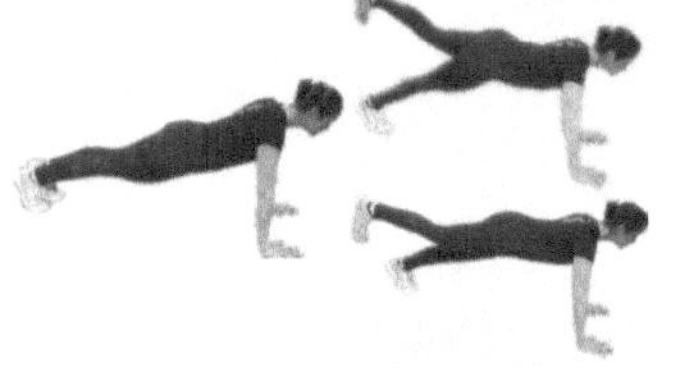

**4** back lunge

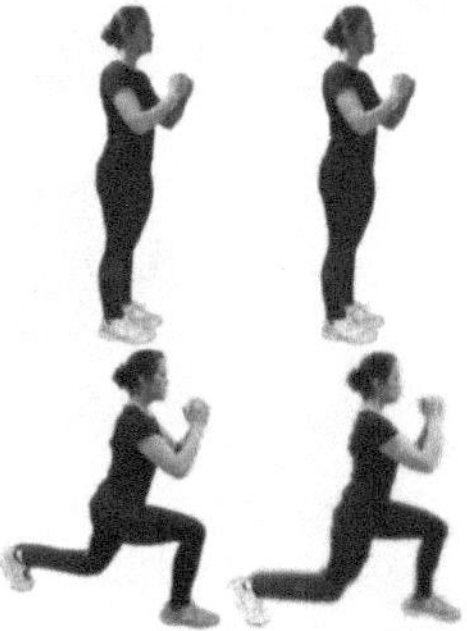

The 6minute clock is continuous. Continue to move through the circuit, performing the repetitions required.

## Cool down – 10 min- see page

Monday Functional High
Intensity Training workout
Week 8

**2 x 7** min
circuits

**14** min
workout time

**37** min
total time

## Warm up -10 min

## F.H.I.T Circuit - 7 min - Repeat 2 times

### 1 squat with hold at bottom

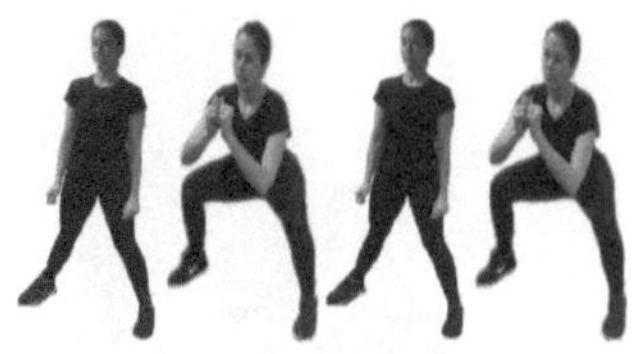

### 2 split jump hold at the bottom

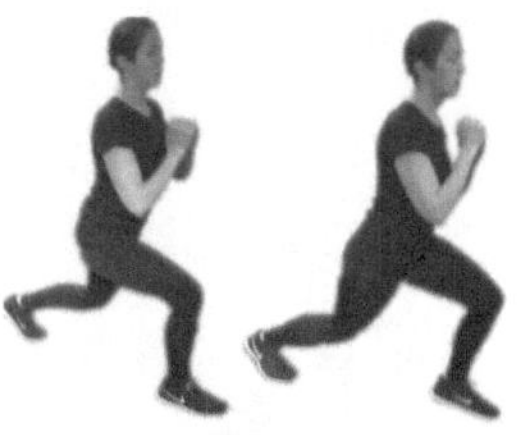

### 3 high knees

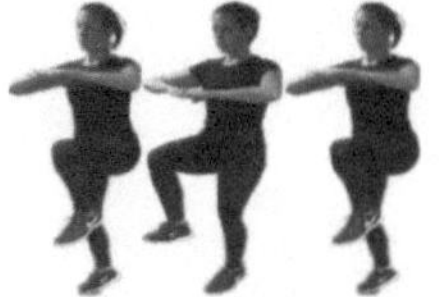

### 4 donkey kick 2sec hold

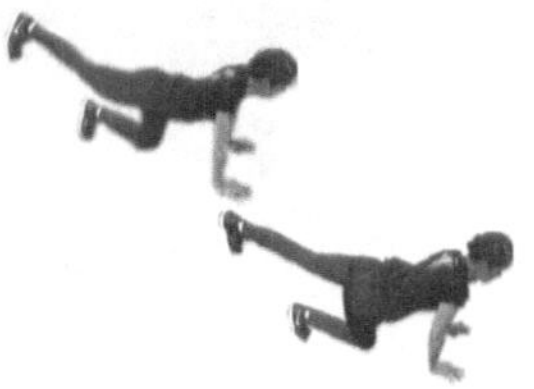

### 5 lateral towel jumps

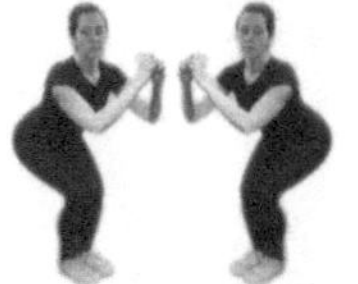

### 6 back lunge hold

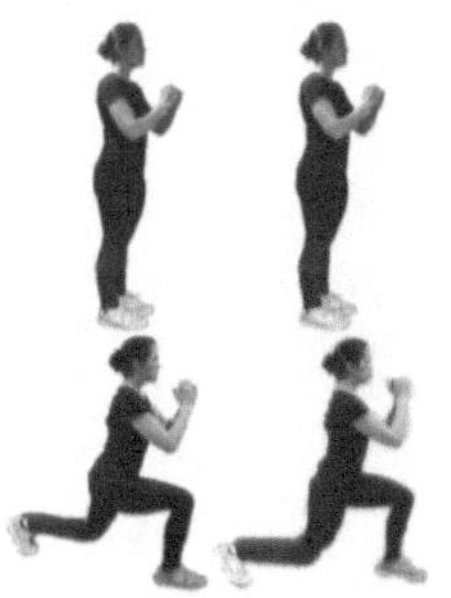

### 7 squat with front kick

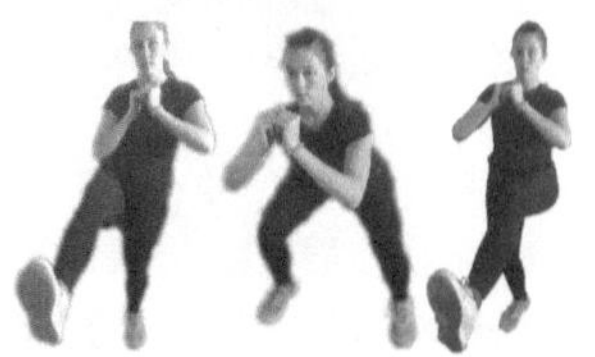

## Rest period between circuit rounds 2 min then begin circuits again.

## Cool down – 10 min- see page

Tuesday is recovery training

Week 8 pre-training

**2 x 5** min
warmup & cool down

**30** min
workout time

**40** min
total time

## Warm up -5 min

## Cardio - 30 min

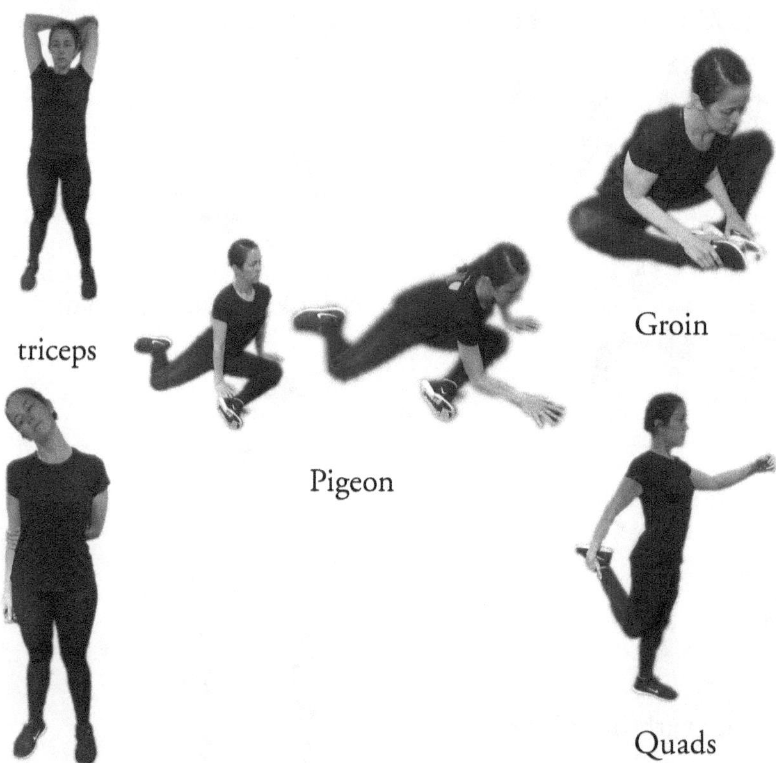

triceps

Pigeon

Groin

Neck & shoulder

Quads

Make sure to follow stretches on page

Cool down – 5 min- see page

Wednesday Functional High Intensity Training workout
Week 8

**2 x 7** min
circuits

**14** min
workout time

**37** min
total time

## Warm up -10 min

## F.H.I.T Circuit - 7 min - Repeat 2 times

1 push up hold

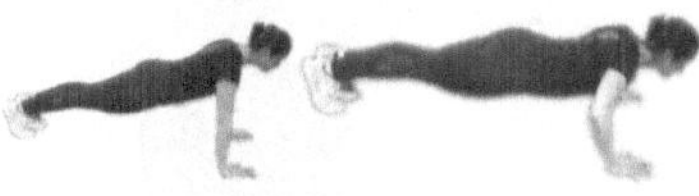

2 v ups

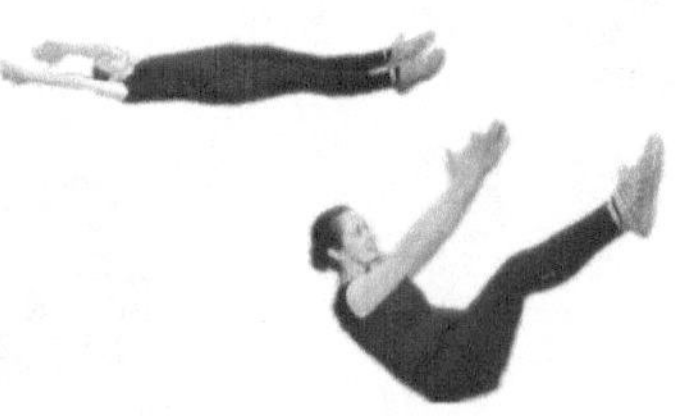

3 mountain climber

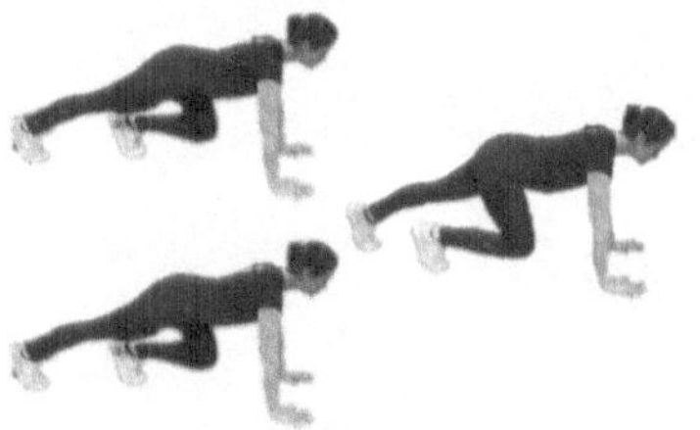

4 superman holds

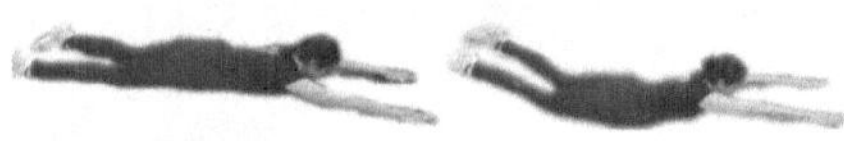

6 bench dips

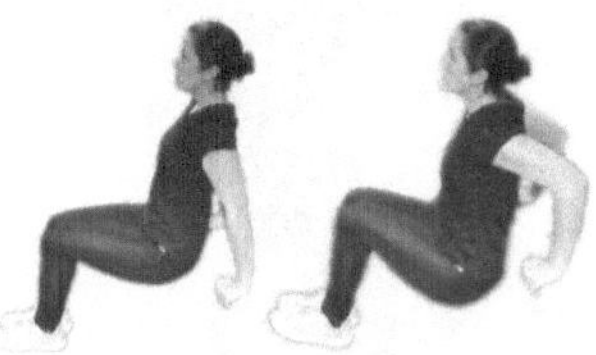

5 plank jacks

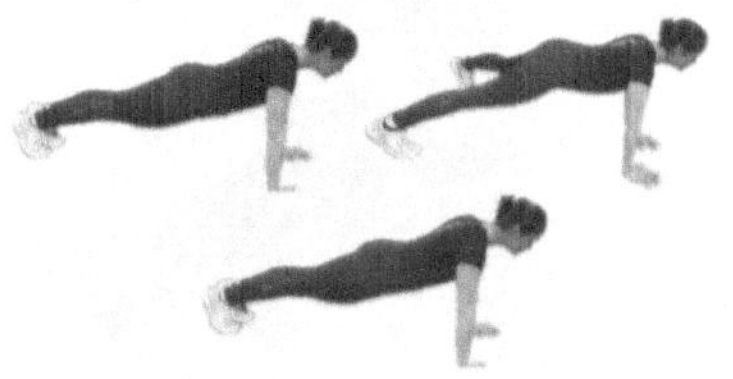

7 bicycle holds

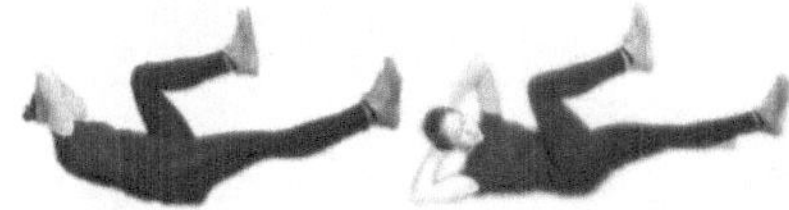

Rest period between circuit rounds 2 min then begin circuits again.

Cool down – 10 min- see page

Thursday Cardio & flexibility training
Week 8 pre-training

**2 x 5** min
warmup & cool down

**30** min
workout time

**40** min
total time

## Warm up -5 min

## Cardio - 30 min

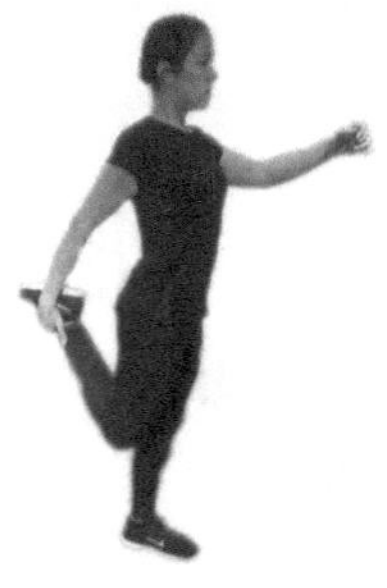

Quad stretch

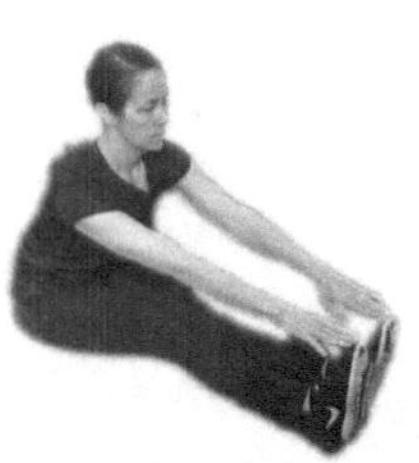

Hamstring stretch

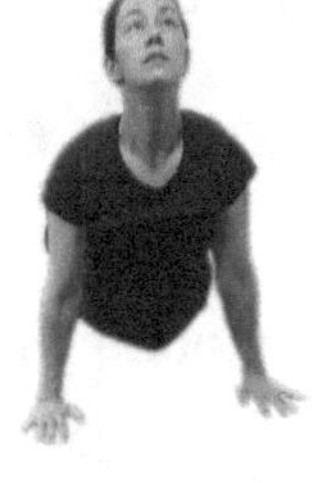

Abdominals

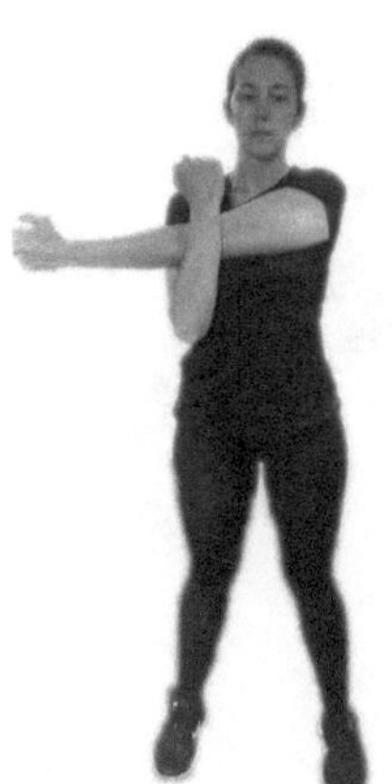

Upper back stretch

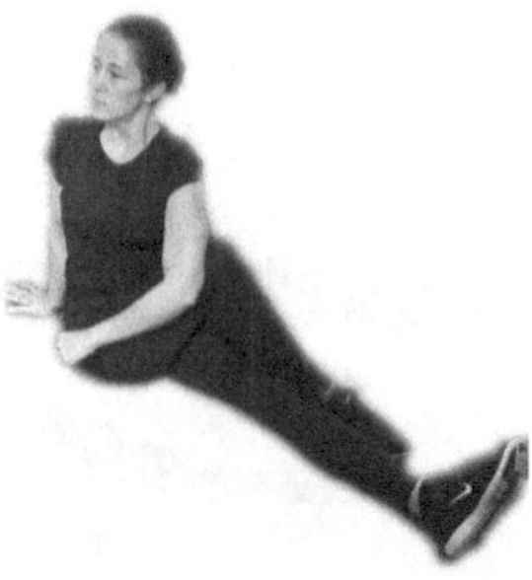

Rotational

## Make sure to follow stretches on page

## Cool down – 5 min- see page

Friday Pioneer Power Training workout
Week 8

**1 x 6** min
circuits

**6** min
workout time

**26** min
total time

## Warm up -10 min

## F.H.I.T Circuit - 7 min - Repeat 2 times

(1) split jumps

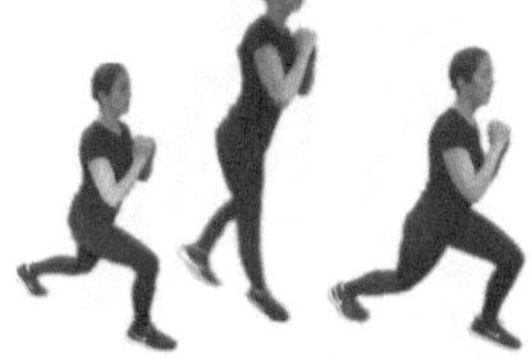

(2) front and back froggers

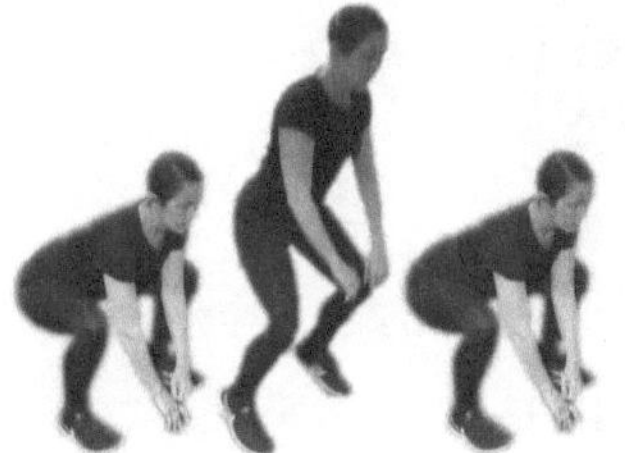

(3) front and back hops

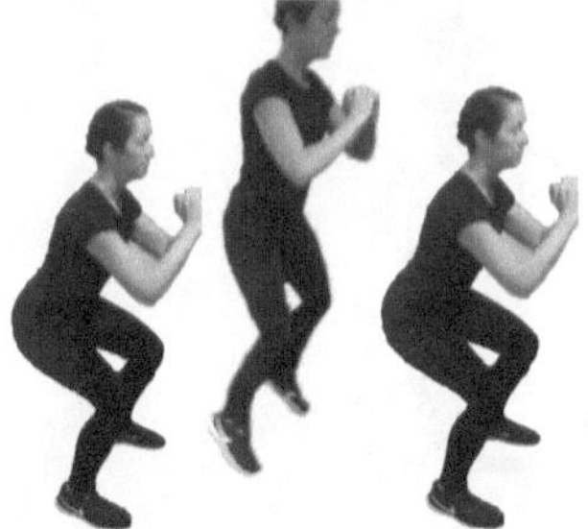

(4) high knees

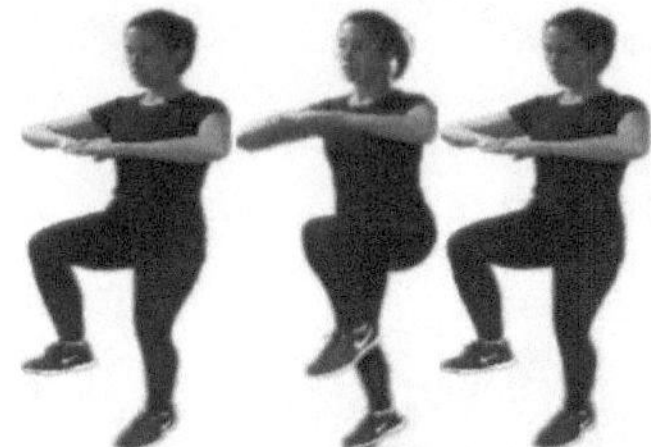

The 6minute clock is continuous. Continue to move through the circuit, performing the repetitions required.

Cool down – 10 min- see page

Monday Functional High
Intensity Training workout
Week 9

**2 x 7** min
circuits

**14** min
workout time

**37** min
total time

## Warm up -10 min

## F.H.I.T Circuit - 7 min - Repeat 2 times

### 1 ski bumps

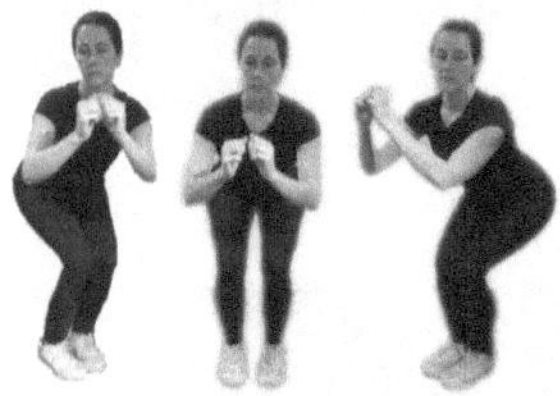

### 2 pioneer in and out squat

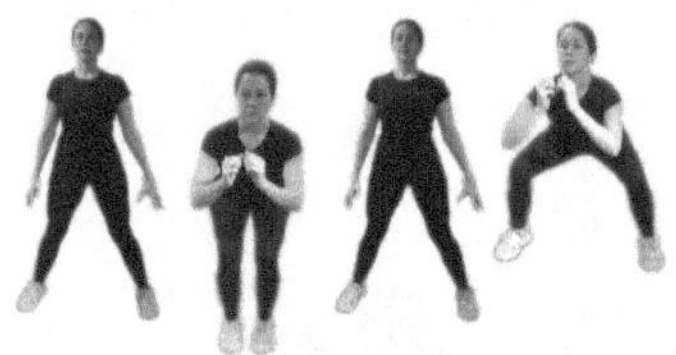

### 3 plank jacks

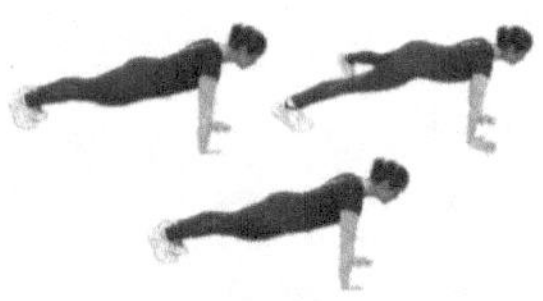

### 4 alternating back lunge

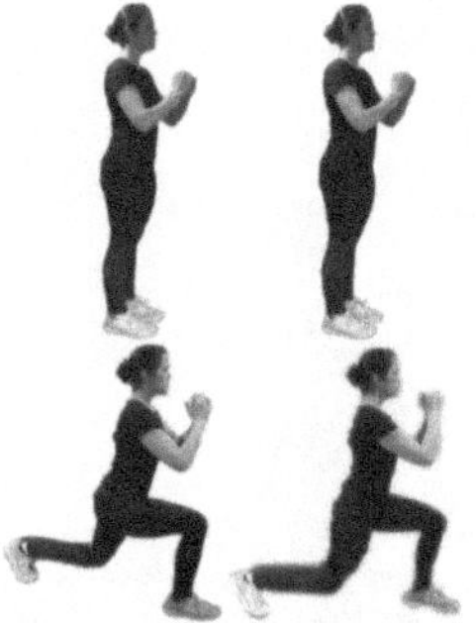

### 5 squat jump

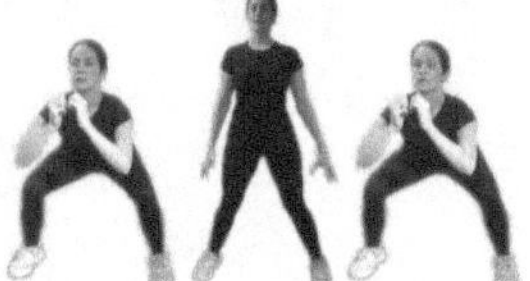

### 6 squat side kick

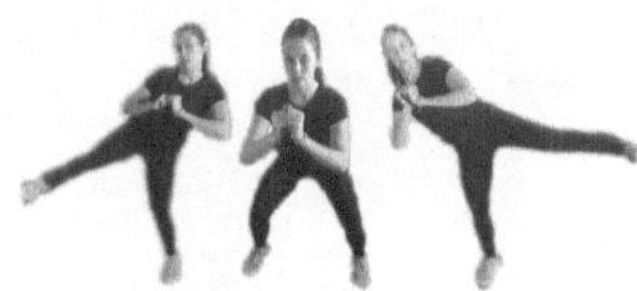

### 7 Leg scissors

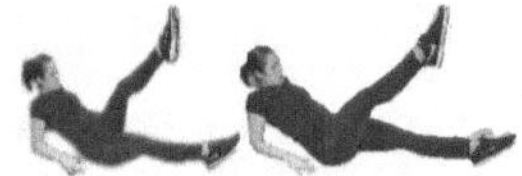

## Rest period between circuit rounds 2 min then begin circuits again.

## Cool down – 10 min- see page

Tuesday is recovery training

Week 9 pre-training

**2 x 5** min
warmup & cool down

**30** min
workout time

**40** min
total time

## Warm up -5 min

## Cardio - 30 min

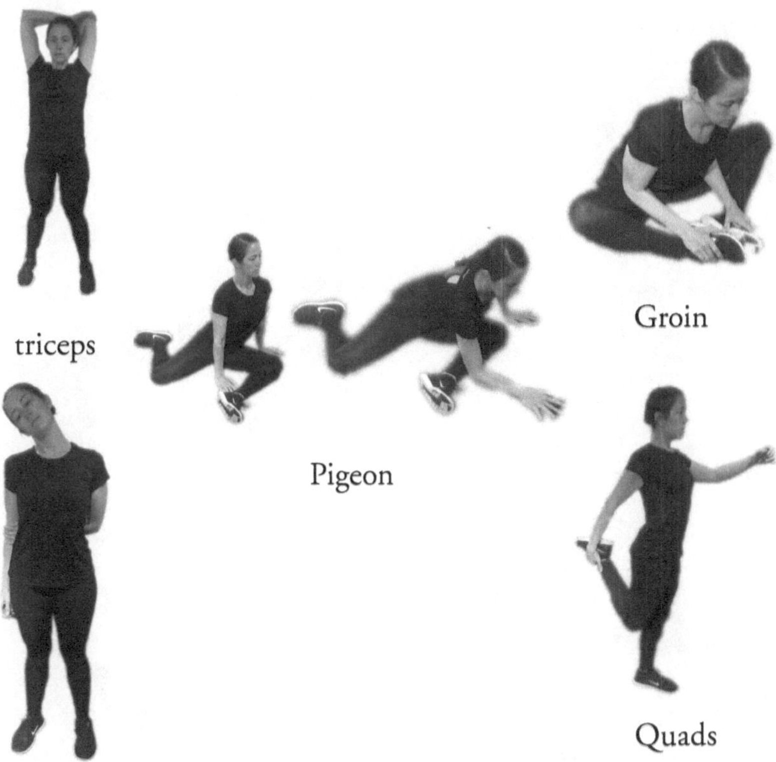

triceps

Groin

Pigeon

Neck & shoulder

Quads

## Make sure to follow stretches on page

## Cool down – 5 min- see page

Wednesday Functional High
Intensity Training workout
Week 9

**2 x 7** min
circuits

**14** min
workout time

**37** min
total time

## Warm up -10 min

## F.H.I.T Circuit - 7 min - Repeat 2 times

### 1 triceps dips

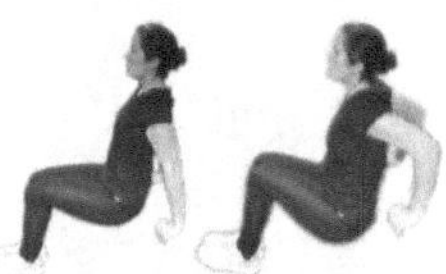

### 2 incline pushup

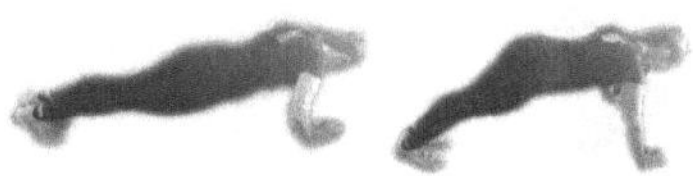

### 3 plank shoulder taps

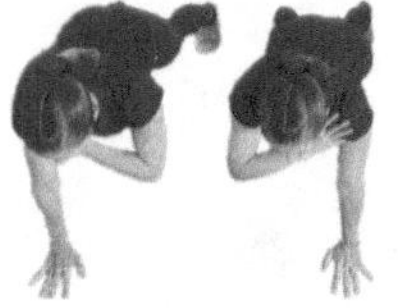

### 4 plank hip rotation

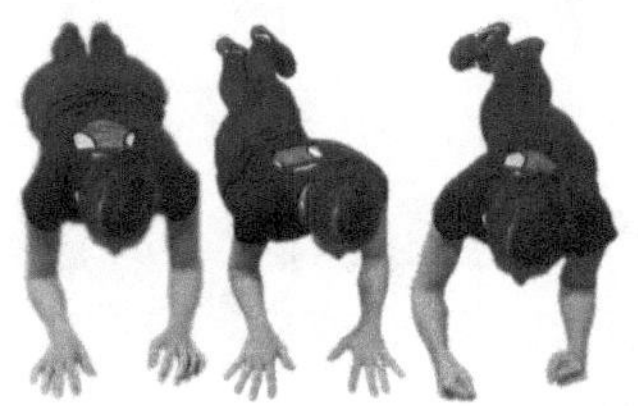

### 5 dive bombers

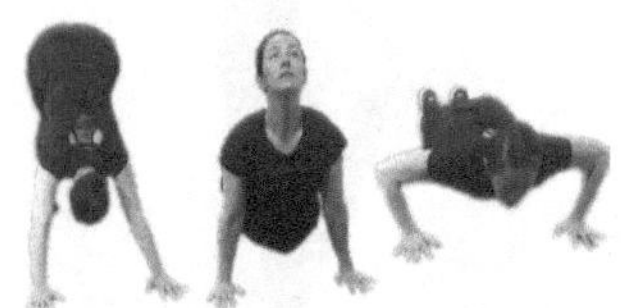

### 6 v ups

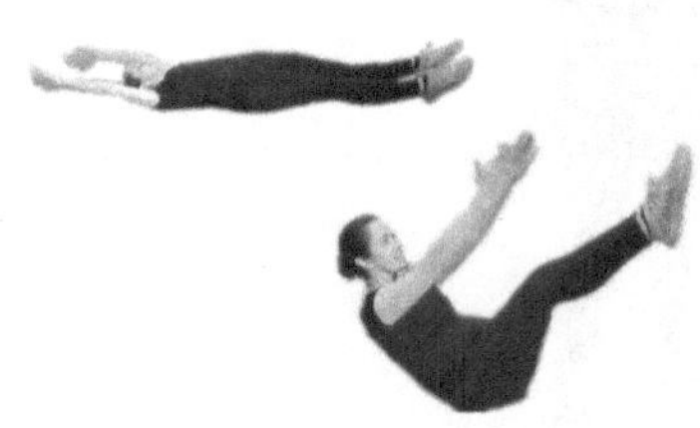

### 7 bungees

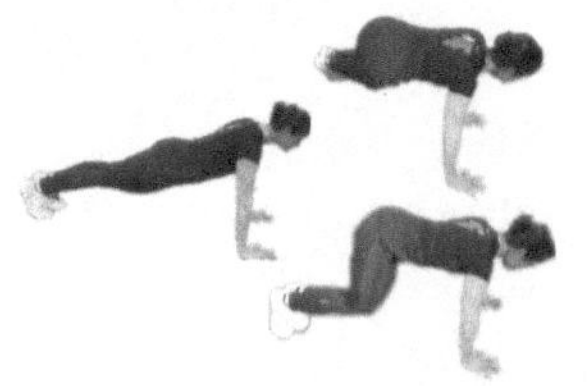

Rest period between circuit rounds 2 min then begin circuits again.

Cool down – 10 min- see page

Thursday Cardio & flexibility training
Week 9 pre-training

**2 x 5** min
warmup & cool down

**30** min
workout time

**40** min
total time

## Warm up -5 min

## Cardio - 30 min

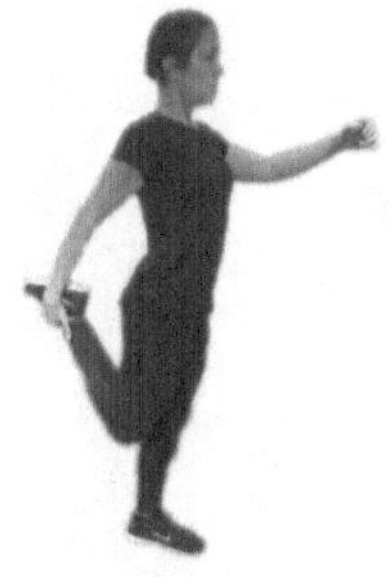

Quad stretch

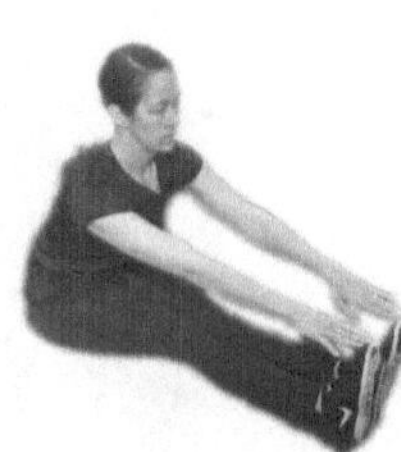

Hamstring stretch

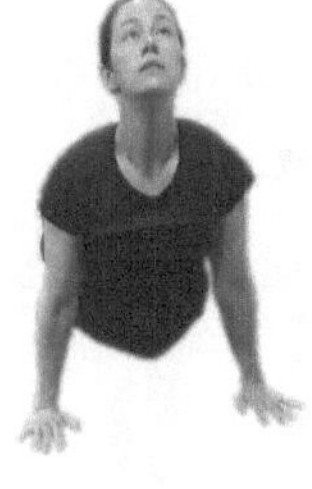

Abdominals

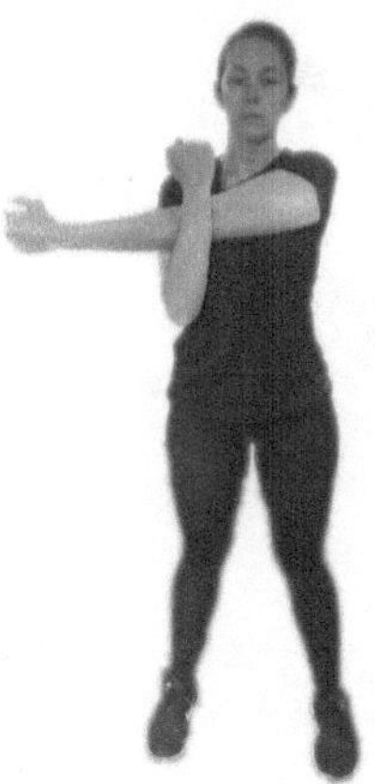

Upper back stretch

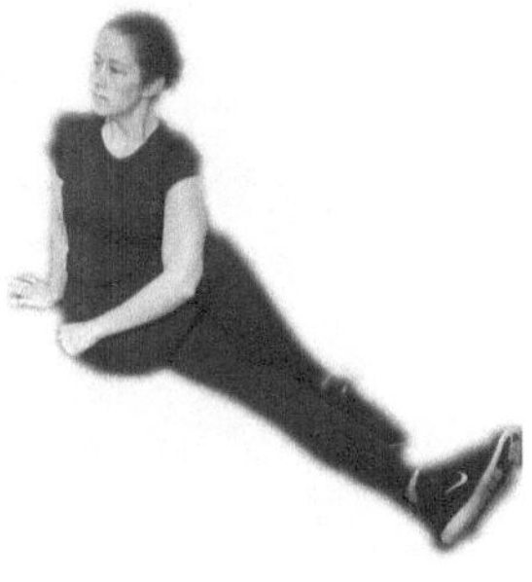

Rotational

## Make sure to follow stretches on page

## Cool down – 5 min- see page

Friday Pioneer Power Training workout
Week 9

**1 x 6**min
circuits

**6**min
workout time

**26**min
total time

## Warm up -10 min

## F.H.I.T Circuit - 7 min - Repeat 2 times

**1** ski bumps

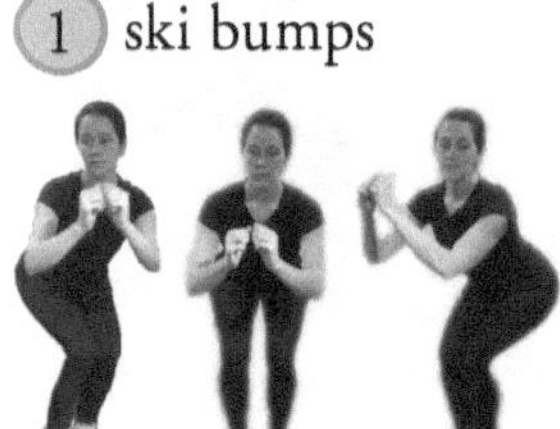

**2** squat front kick

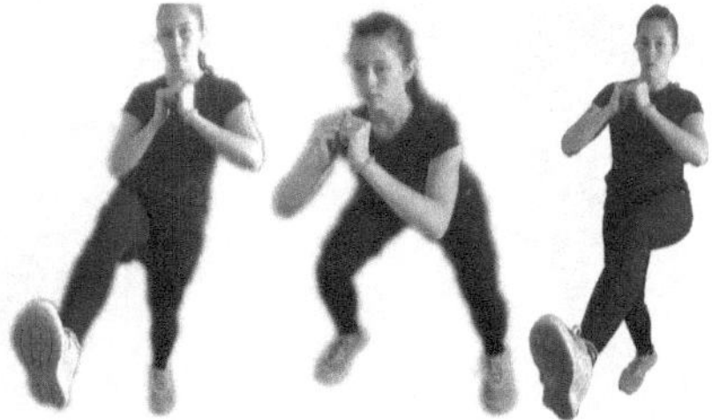

**3** burpee

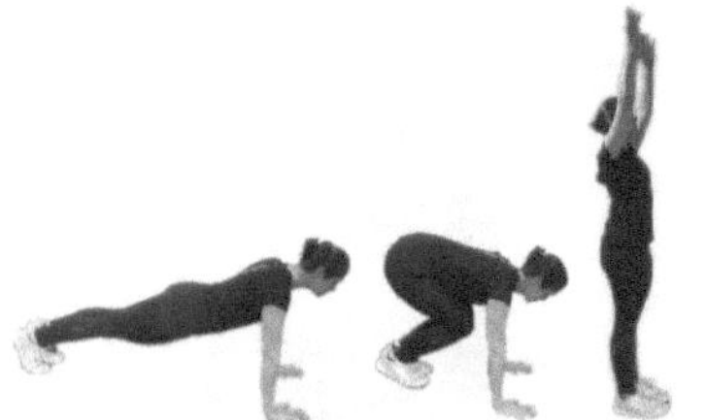

**4** mountain climbers

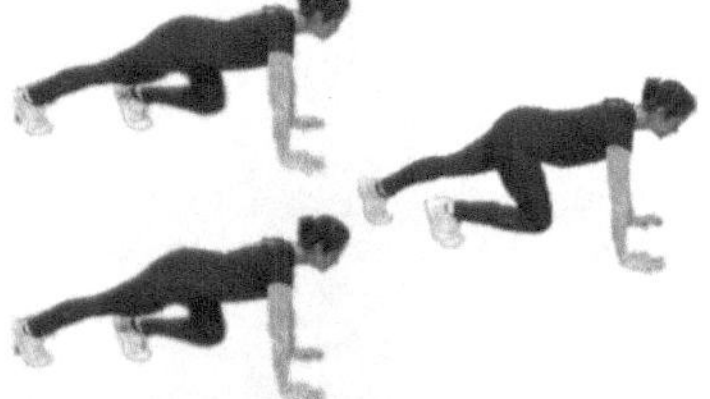

The 6minute clock is continuous. Continue to move through the circuit, performing the repetitions required.

## Cool down – 10 min- see page

Monday Functional High
Intensity Training workout
Week 10

**2 x 7** min
circuits

**14** min
workout time

**37** min
total time

## Warm up -10 min

## F.H.I.T Circuit - 7 min - Repeat 2 times

### 1 front and back froggers

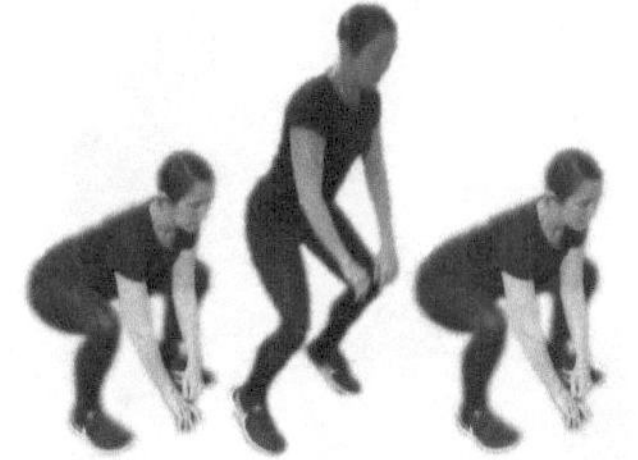

### 2 lateral lunge

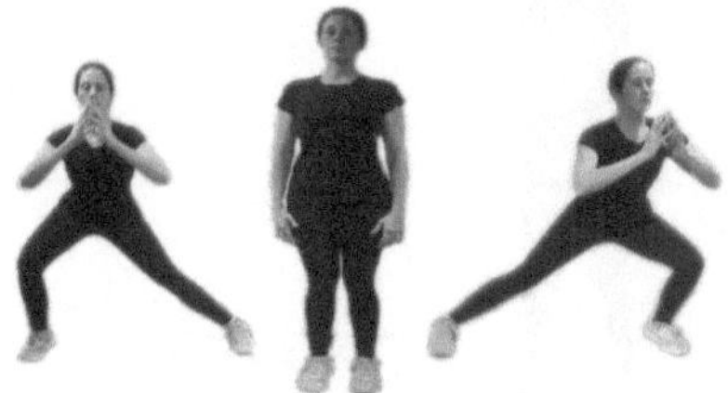

### 3 squat front kick

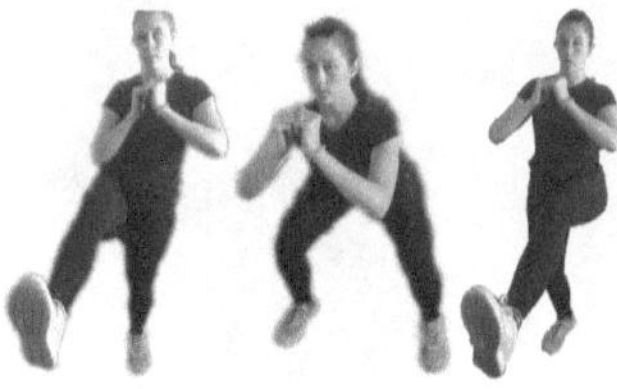

### 4 plank jacks

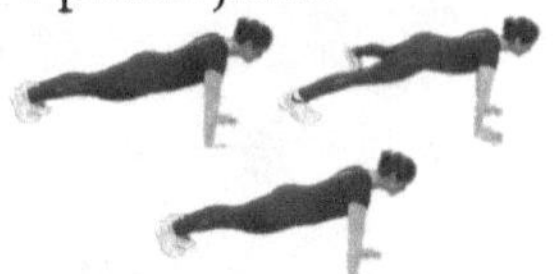

### 6 glute bridges

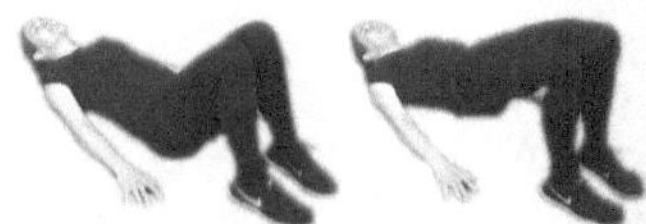

### 5 half burpees

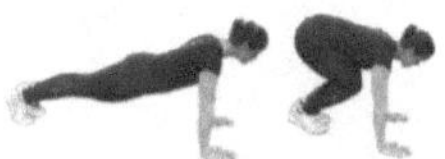

### 7 high knee

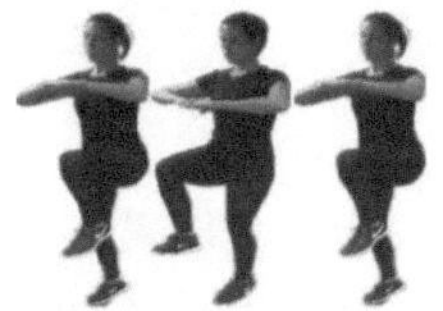

Rest period between circuit rounds 2 min then begin circuits again.

Cool down – 10 min- see page

Tuesday is recovery training

Week 10 pre-training

**2 x 5** min
warmup & cool down

**30** min
workout time

**40** min
total time

## Warm up -5 min

## Cardio - 30 min

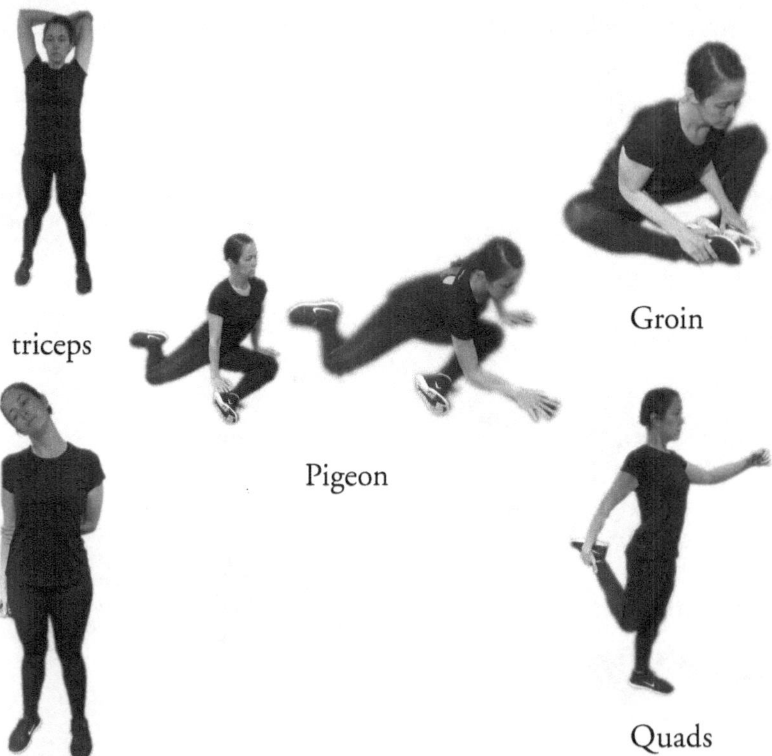


## Make sure to follow stretches on page

## Cool down – 5 min- see page

Wednesday Functional High
Intensity Training workout
Week 10

**2 x 7** min
circuits

**14** min
workout time

**37** min
total time

## Warm up -10 min

## F.H.I.T Circuit - 7 min - Repeat 2 times

### 1 power jumps

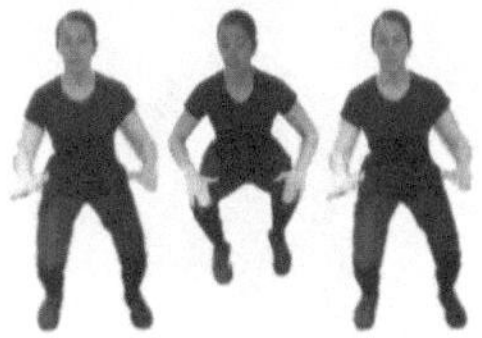

### 2 alternating front lunge

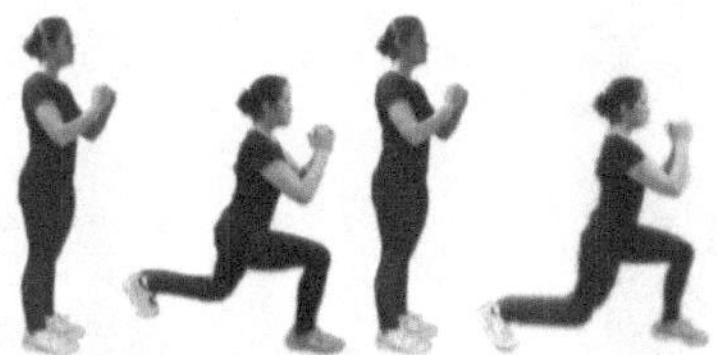

### 3 half burpees

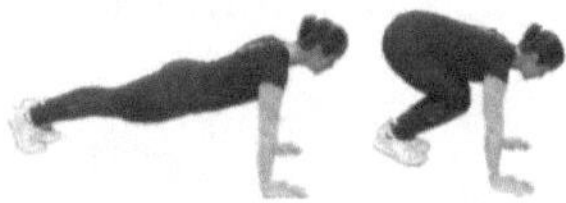

### 4 pioneer squats in and out

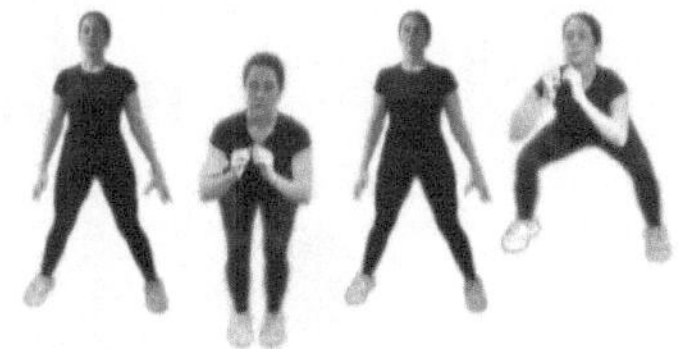

### 5 bungee

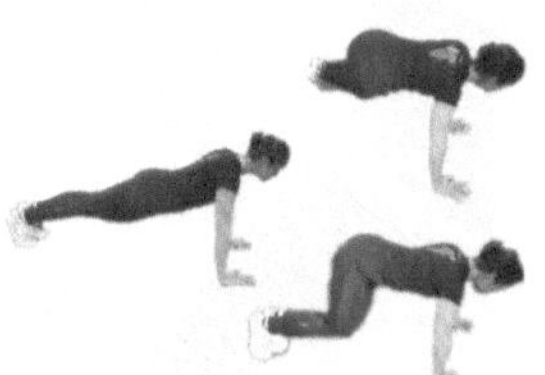

### 6 alternating limb lifts

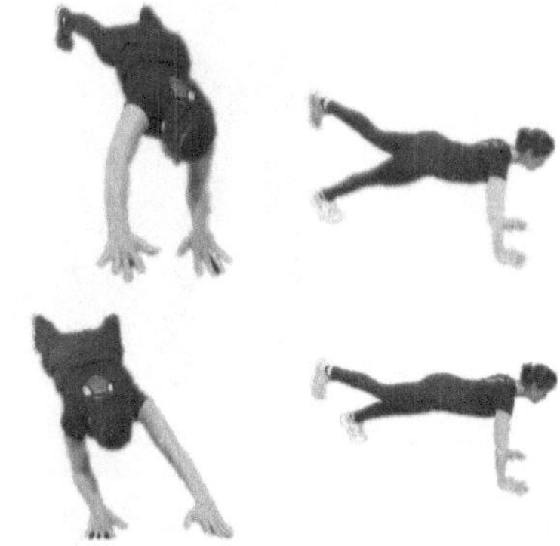

### 7 plank rotation

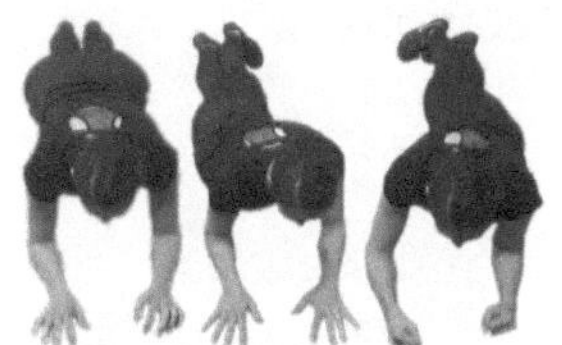

## Rest period between circuit rounds 2 min then begin circuits again.

## Cool down – 10 min- see page

Thursday Cardio & flexibility training
Week 10 pre-training

**2 x 5** min
warmup & cool down

**30** min
workout time

**40** min
total time

## Warm up -5 min

## Cardio - 30 min

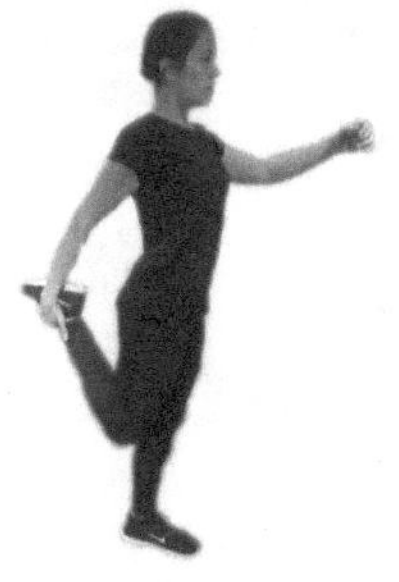

Quad stretch

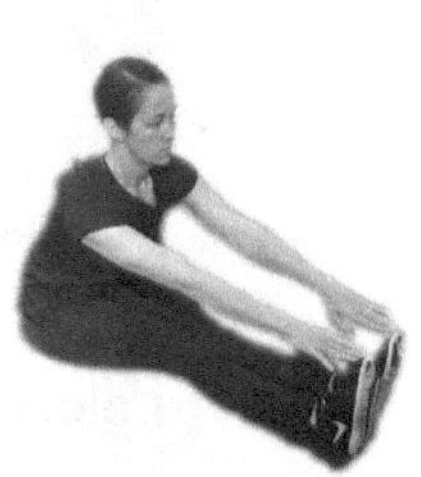

Hamstring stretch

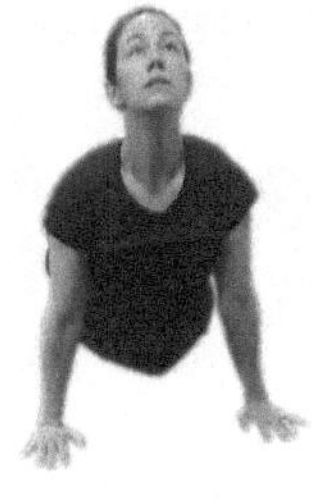

Abdominals

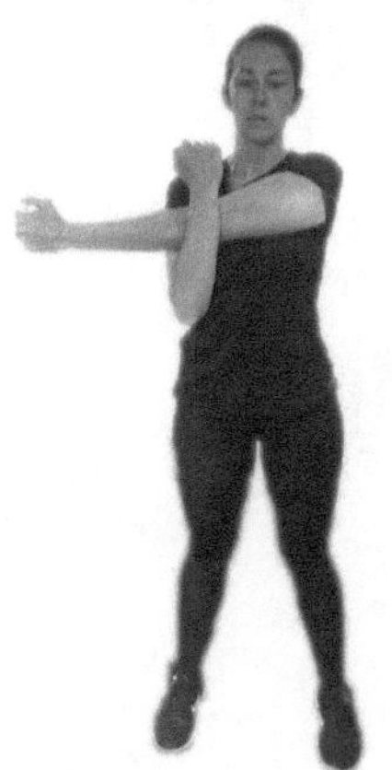

Upper back stretch

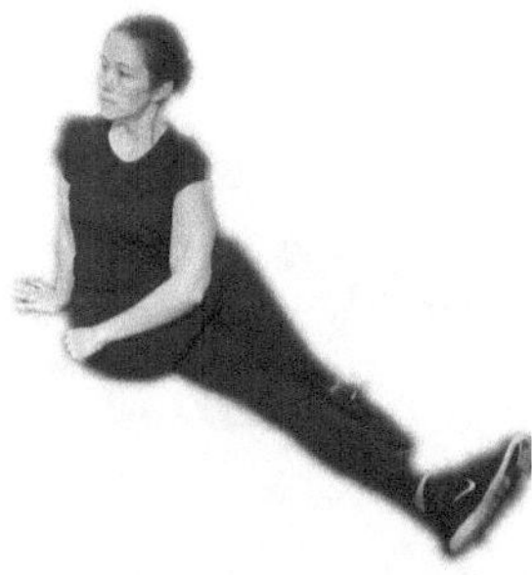

Rotational

## Make sure to follow stretches on page

## Cool down – 5 min- see page

Friday Pioneer Power Training workout
Week 10

**1 x 6** min
circuits

**6** min
workout time

**26** min
total time

## Warm up -10 min

## F.H.I.T Circuit - 7 min - Repeat 2 times

(1) triceps dips

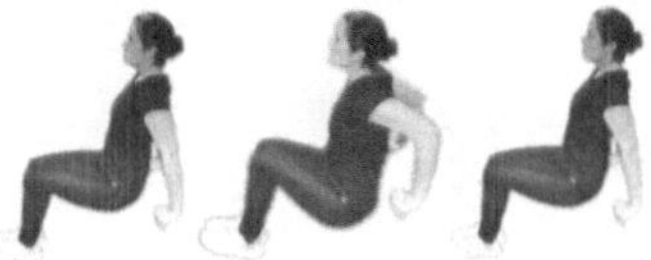

(3) dive bombers

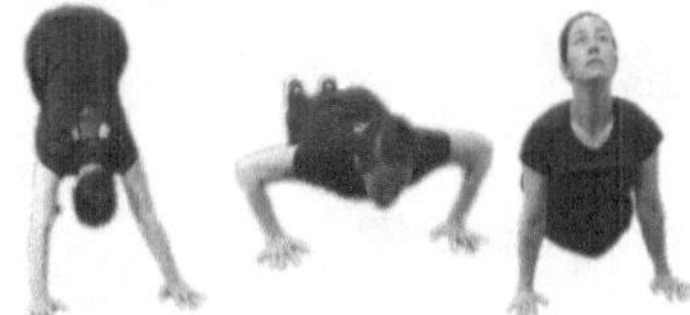

(2) wide pushups

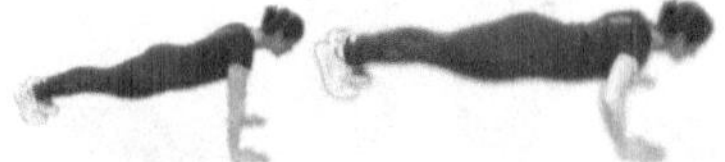

(4) bicycles

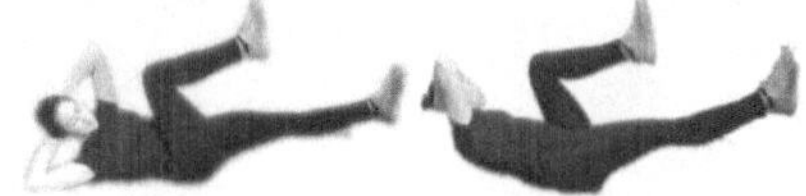

The 6minute clock is continuous. Continue to move through the circuit, performing the repetitions required.

## Cool down – 10 min- see page

Monday Functional High
Intensity Training workout
Week 11

**2 x 7** min
circuits

**14** min
workout time

**37** min
total time

## Warm up -10 min

## F.H.I.T Circuit - 7 min - Repeat 2 times

### 1 lateral shuffle

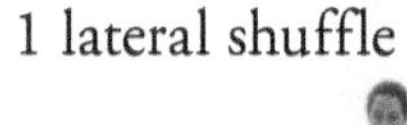

### 2 switch kicks

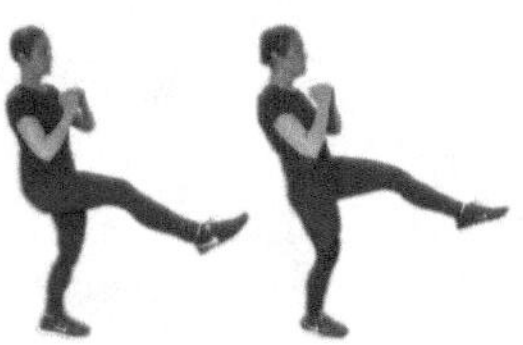

### 3 split jumps

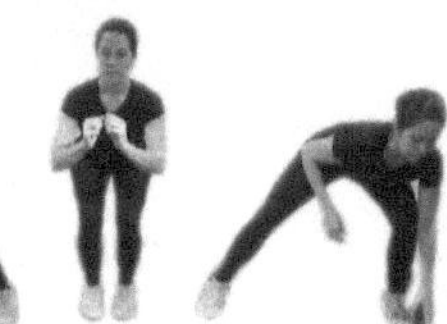

### 4 plank jacks

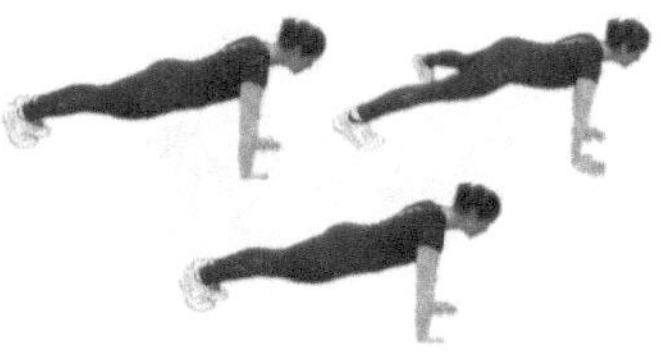

### 5 2 push up and move

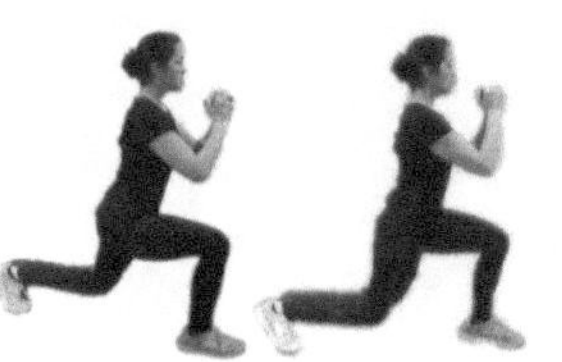

### 6 squat touch turns

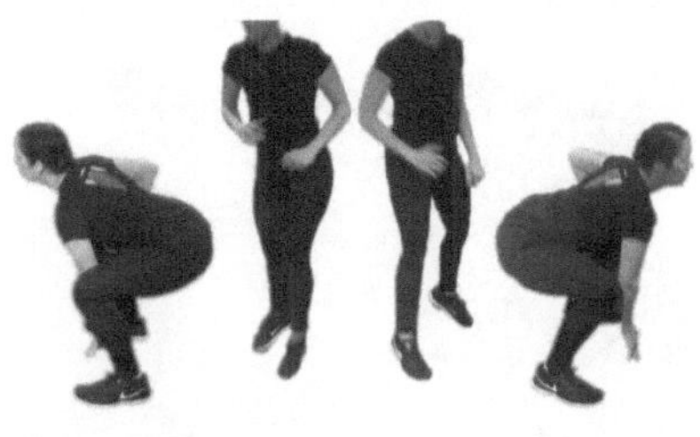

### 7 robot pushups

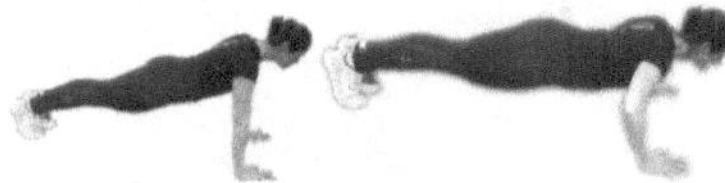
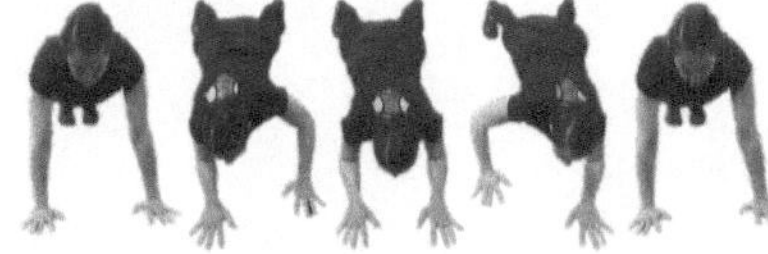

Rest period between circuit rounds 2 min then begin circuits again.

Cool down – 10 min- see page

Tuesday is recovery training

Week 11 pre-training

**2 x 5** min
warmup & cool down

**30** min
workout time

**40** min
total time

## Warm up -5 min

## Cardio - 30 min

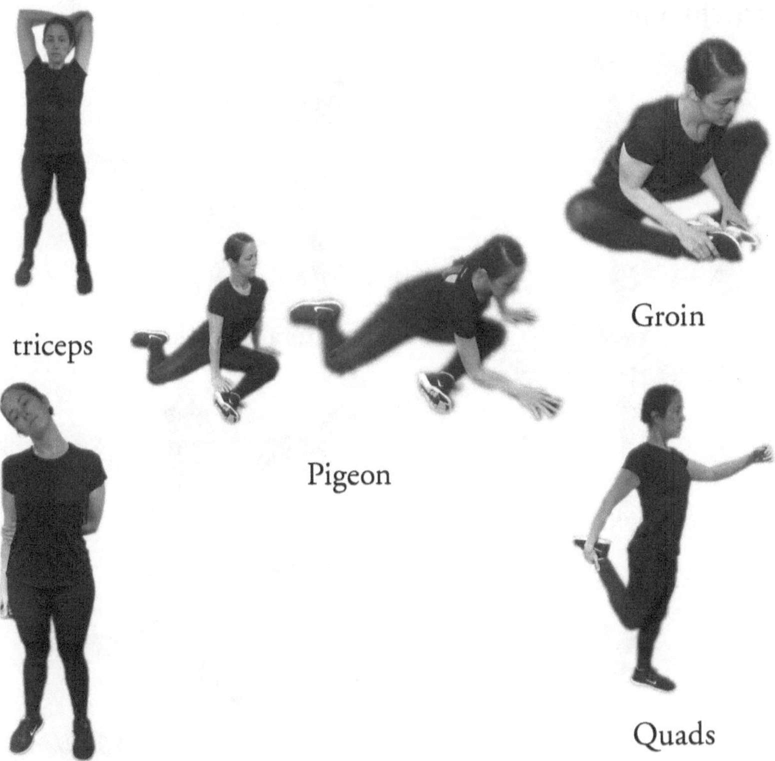


Make sure to follow stretches on page

Cool down – 5 min- see page

Wednesday Functional High
Intensity Training workout
Week 11

**2 x 7** min
circuits

**14** min
workout time

**37** min
total time

## Warm up -10 min

## F.H.I.T Circuit - 7 min - Repeat 2 times

### 1 triceps dips
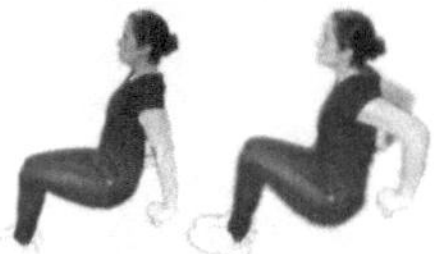

### 2 switch kicks
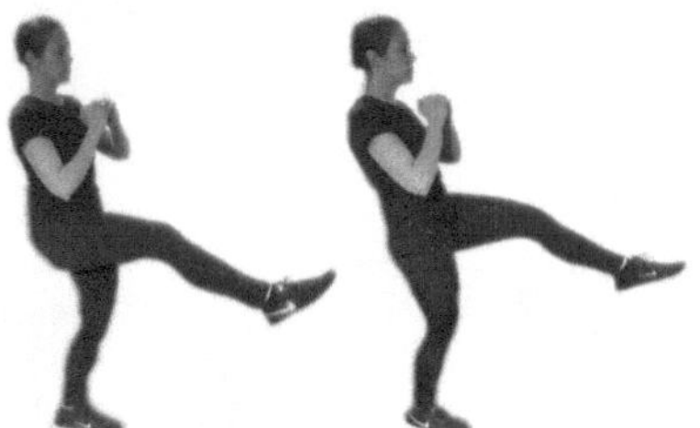

### 3 123 knee
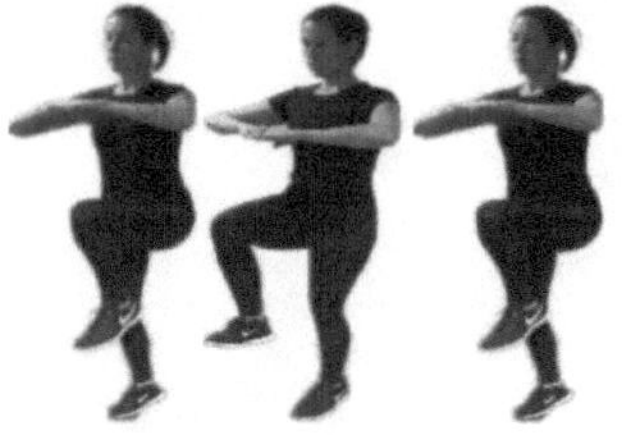

### 4 lateral shuffles
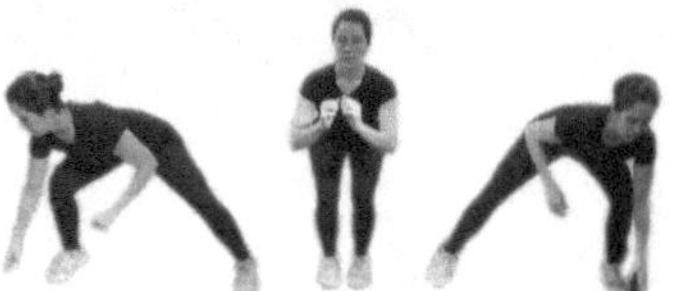

### 5 push up jacks
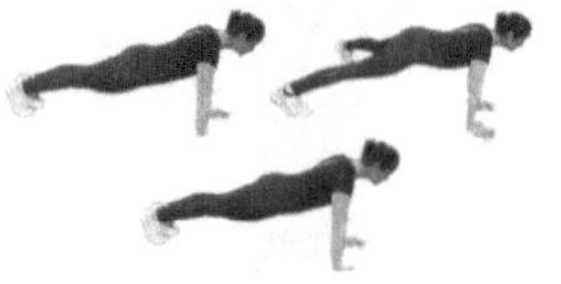

### 6 plank alternating leg lifts
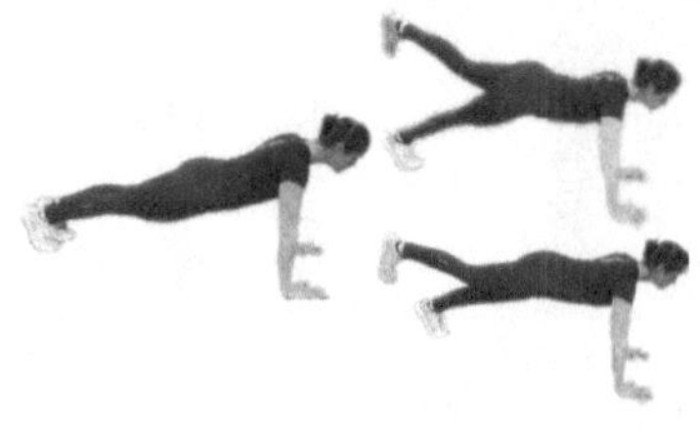

### 7 bicycles
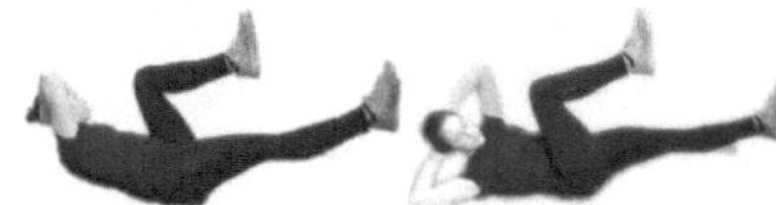

Rest period between circuit rounds 2 min then begin circuits again.

Cool down – 10 min- see page

Thursday Cardio & flexibility training
Week 11 pre-training

**2 x 5** min
warmup & cool down

**30**min
workout time

**40**min
total time

## Warm up -5 min

## Cardio - 30 min

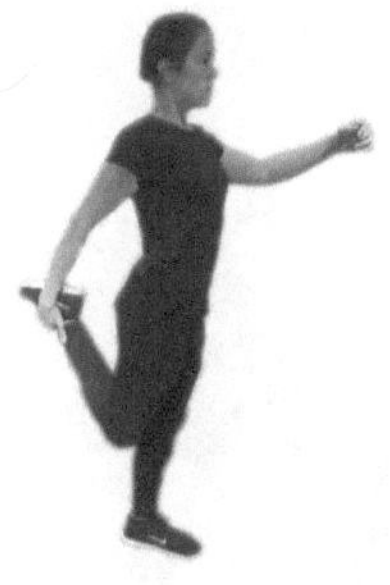

Quad stretch

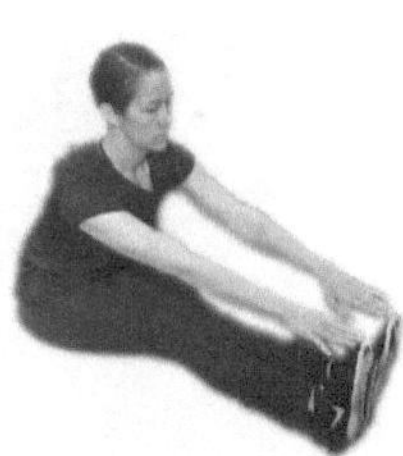

Hamstring stretch

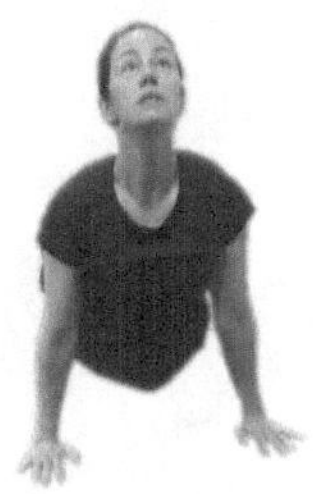

Abdominals

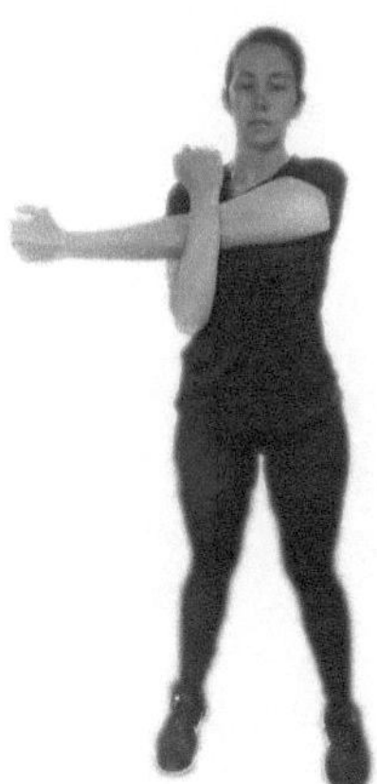

Upper back stretch

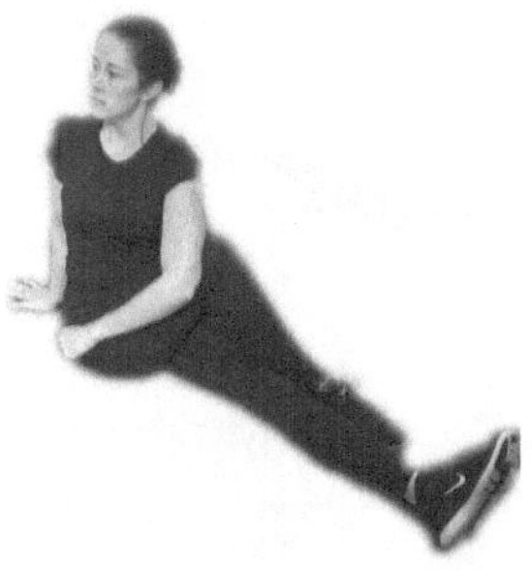

Rotational

## Make sure to follow stretches on page

## Cool down – 5 min- see page

Friday Pioneer Power Training
workout
Week 11

## 1 x 6 min
circuits

## 6 min
workout time

## 26 min
total time

---

## Warm up -10 min

## F.H.I.T Circuit - 7 min - Repeat 2 times

**1** lateral lunge

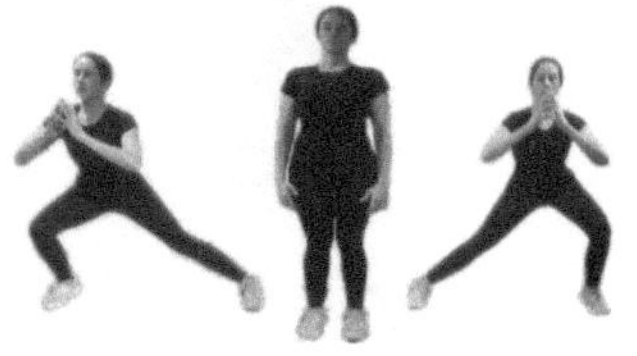

**4** plank rotation

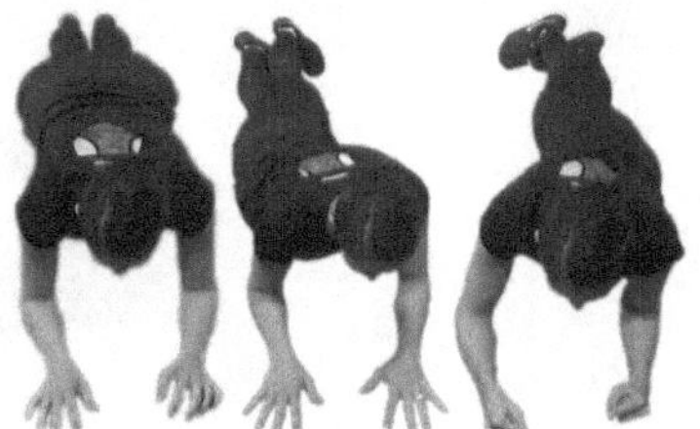

**3** burpees

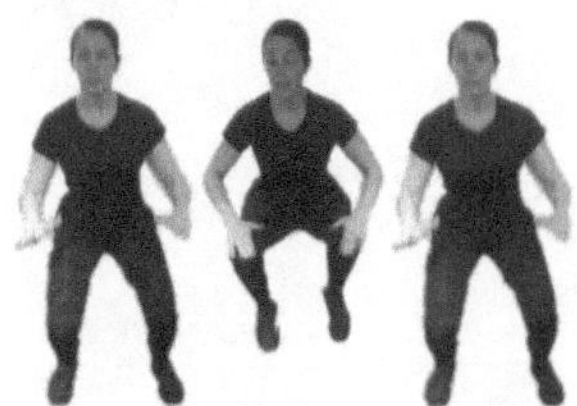

**2** power jumps

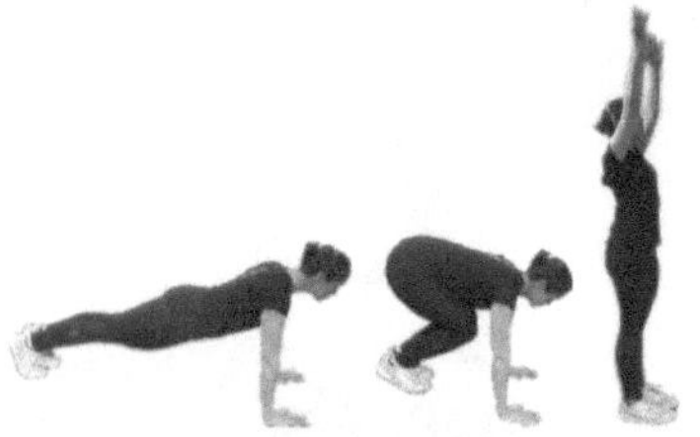

The 6minute clock is continuous. Continue to move through the circuit, performing the repetitions required.

Cool down – 10 min- see page

---

Monday Functional High
Intensity Training workout
Week 12

**2 x 7** min
circuits

**14** min
workout time

**37** min
total time

## Warm up -10 min

## F.H.I.T Circuit - 7 min - Repeat 2 times

1 front and back hops

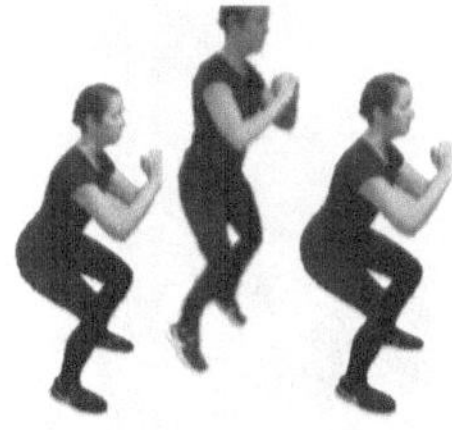

3 squats with side kicks

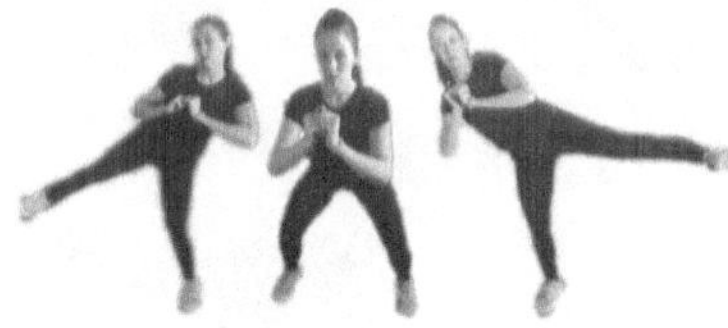

5 bungees

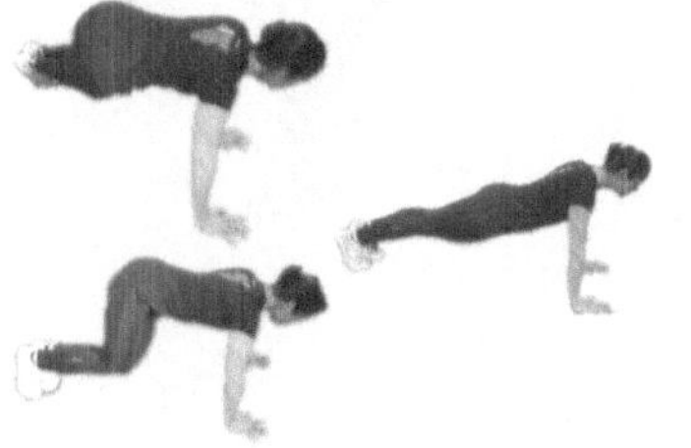

7 high knees

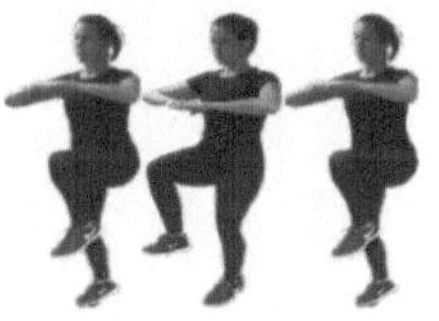

2 lateral lunges

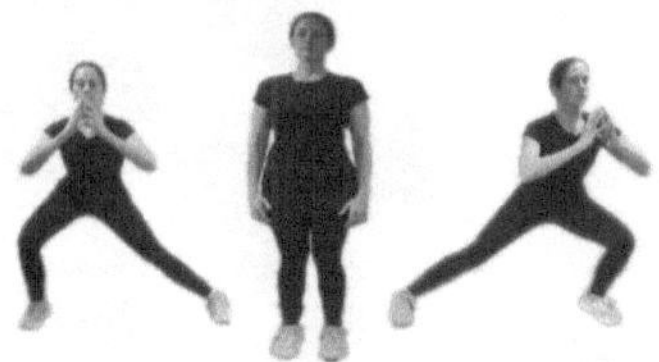

4 plank jacks

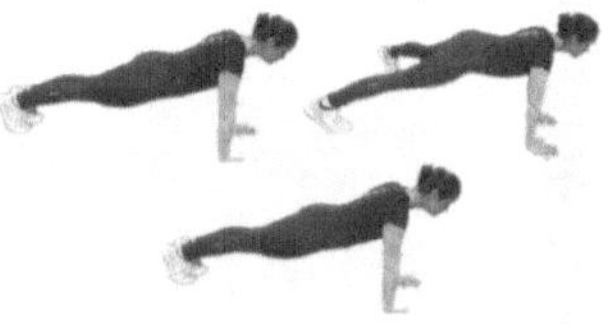

6 glute bridges

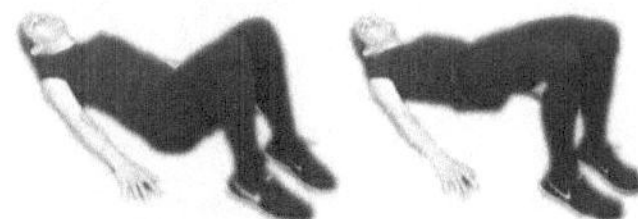

## Rest period between circuit rounds 2 min then begin circuits again.

## Cool down – 10 min- see page

Tuesday is recovery training

Week 11 pre-training

**2 x 5** min
warmup & cool down

**30** min
workout time

**40** min
total time

## Warm up -5 min

## Cardio - 30 min

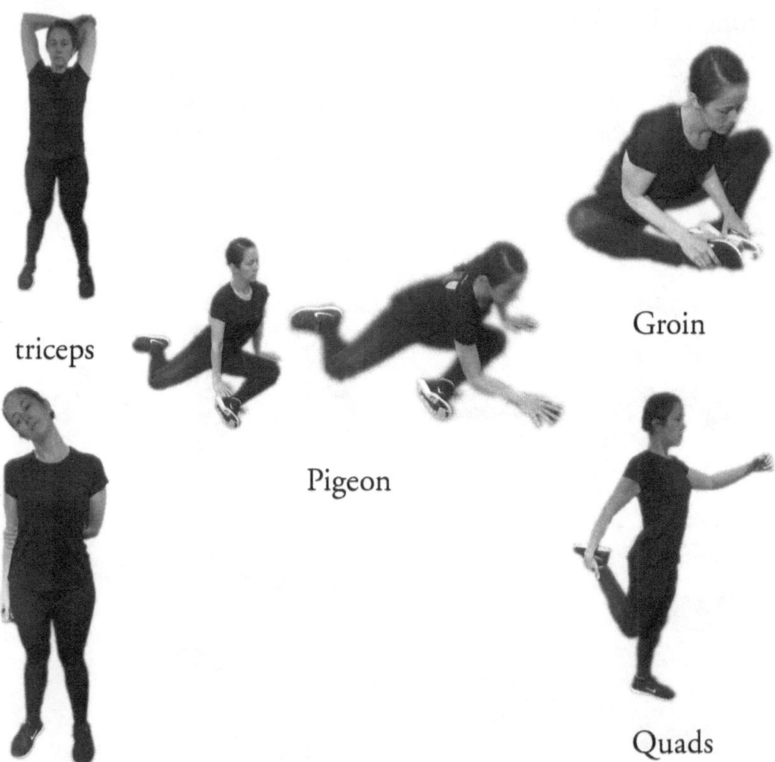


## Make sure to follow stretches on page

## Cool down – 5 min- see page

Wednesday Functional High
Intensity Training workout
Week 12

**2 x 7** min
circuits

**14** min
workout time

**37** min
total time



## F.H.I.T Circuit - 7 min - Repeat 2 times

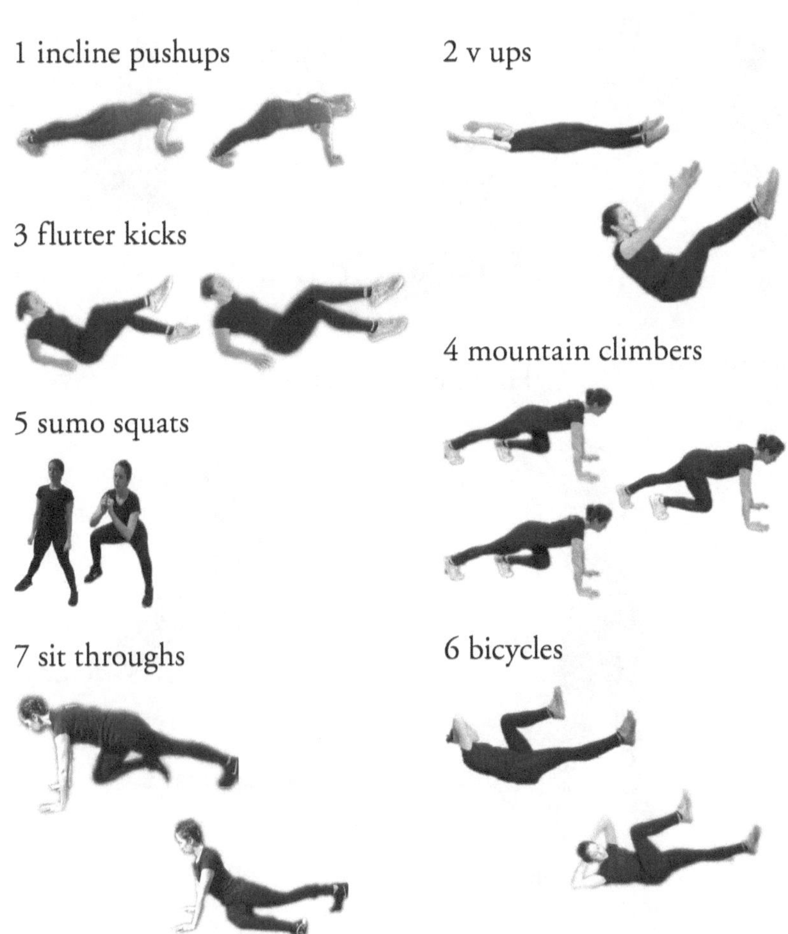

1 incline pushups

2 v ups

3 flutter kicks

4 mountain climbers

5 sumo squats

7 sit throughs

6 bicycles

Rest period between circuit rounds 2 min then begin circuits again.

Cool down – 10 min- see page

Thursday Cardio & flexibility training
Week 12 pre-training

**2 x 5** min
warmup & cool down

**30** min
workout time

**40** min
total time

## Warm up -5 min

## Cardio - 30 min

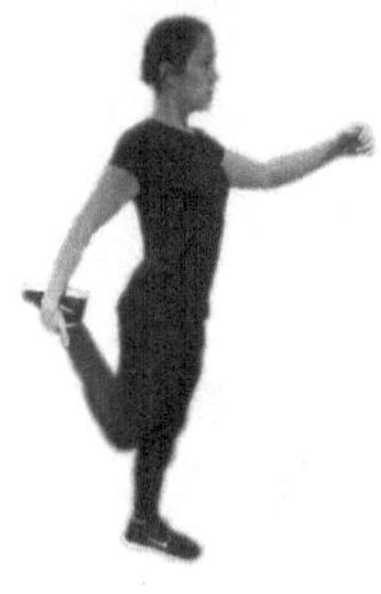

Quad stretch

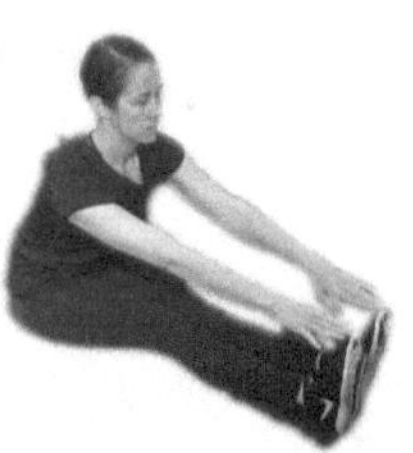

Hamstring stretch

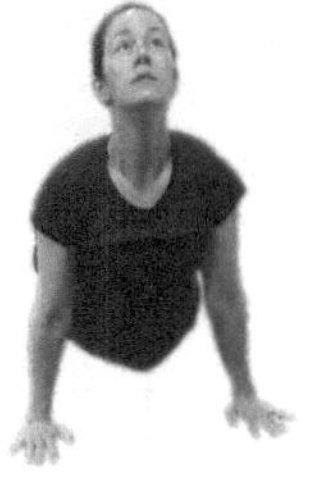

Abdominals

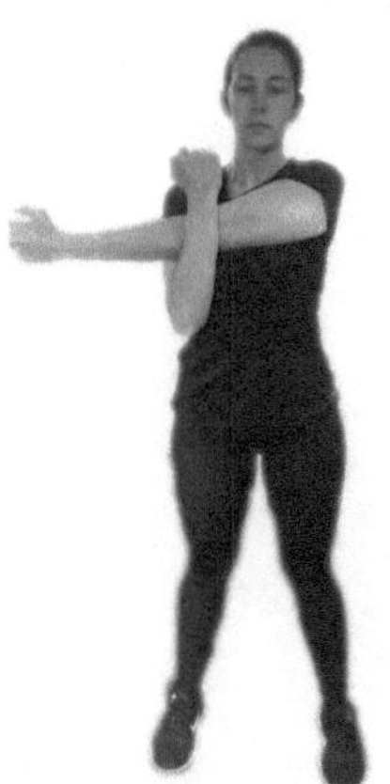

Upper back stretch

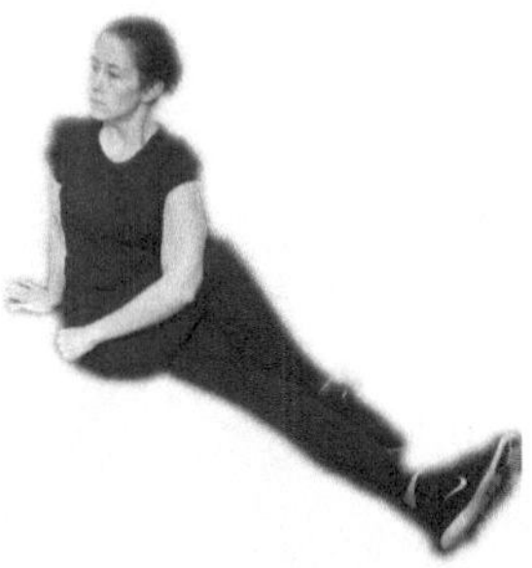

Rotational

## Make sure to follow stretches on page

## Cool down – 5 min- see page

Friday Pioneer Power Training workout
Week 12

**1 x 6** min
circuits

**6** min
workout time

**26** min
total time

## Warm up -10 min

## F.H.I.T Circuit - 7 min - Repeat 2 times

1 split jumps

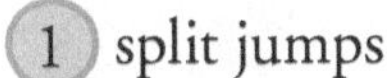
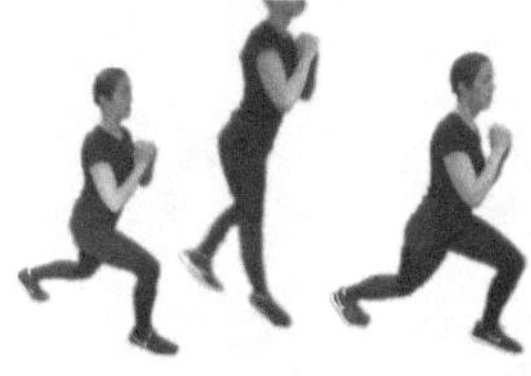

3 plank alternating leg lift

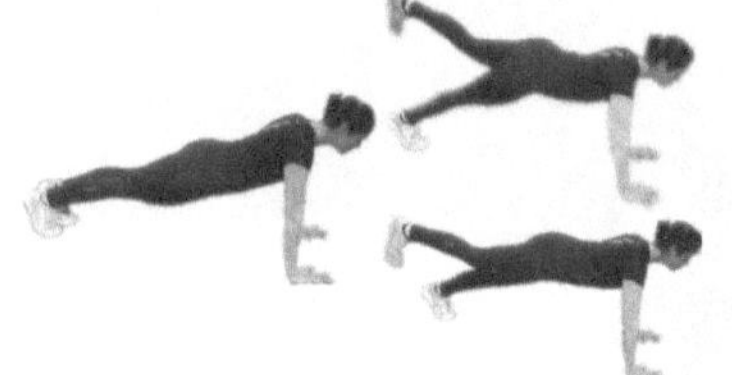

2 v ups

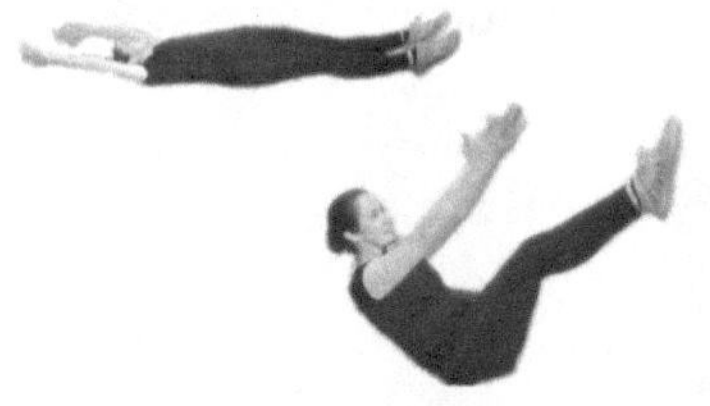

4 back lunge

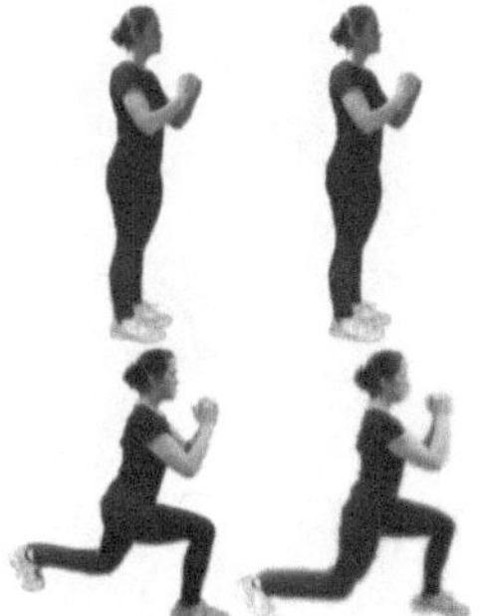

The 6minute clock is continuous. Continue to move through the circuit, performing the repetitions required.

## Cool down – 10 min- see page

Cool down
Week 1

# STRETCHES

**10**min
total time

## Warm up -4 min JOG OR WALK

## COOL DOWN STRETCHES – 6 MINUTES

Hamstring

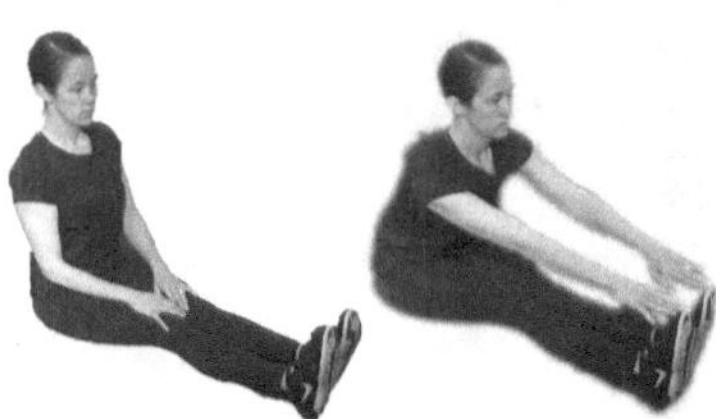

Upper back/ Rear Delt

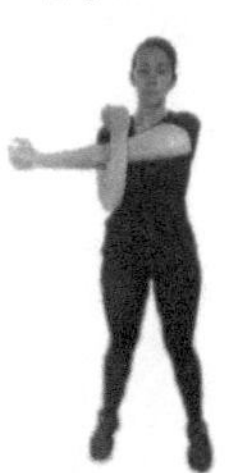

Quadricep/ hip flexor

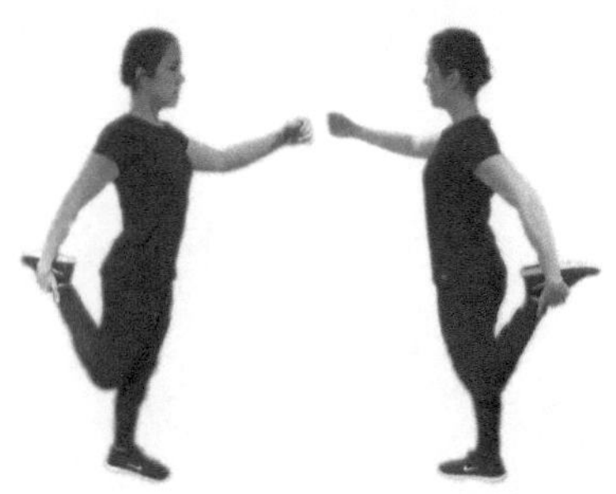

Triceps stretch

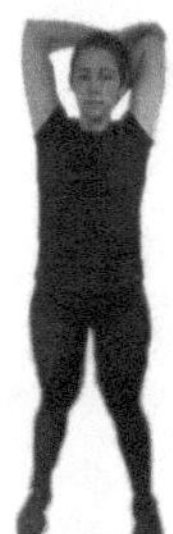

Neck/ Shoulder

Modified Pigeon

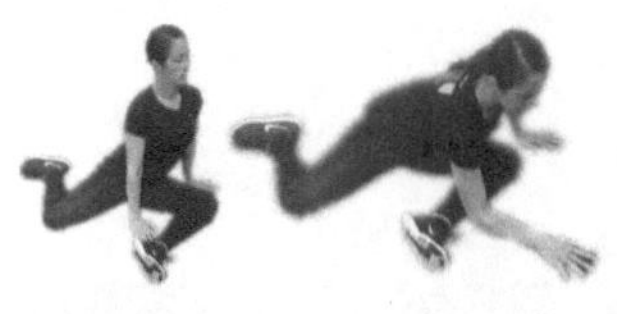

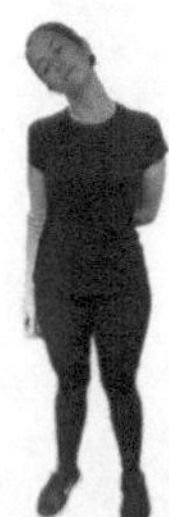

## CORE TRAINING – 5 min- see page

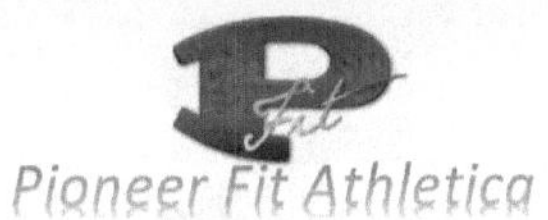
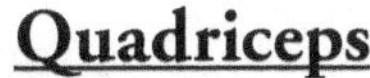


## <u>Quadriceps</u>

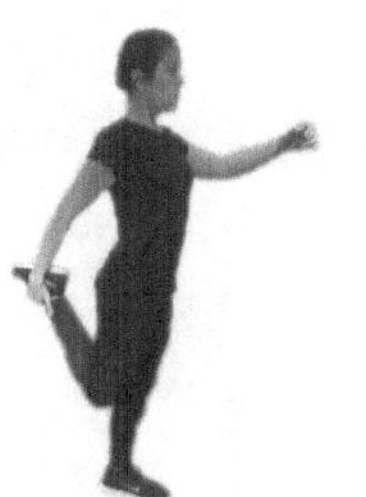

- Standing straight, shift your bodyweight onto your left leg.
- Bring your right foot as close to your glute as possible, try to hold for 20-30 sec.
- Repeat with your left leg.

## <u>Rear Delt /Upper Back</u>

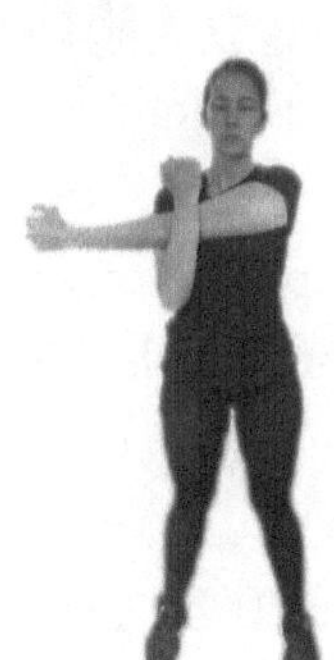

- Standing with feet shoulder width apart.
- Keep your left arm straight and bring it across your chest. Bend your right elbow upwards, brining your right hand even closer to your chest.
- Holding for 20-30 seconds and repeat with other side.

## <u>Triceps</u>

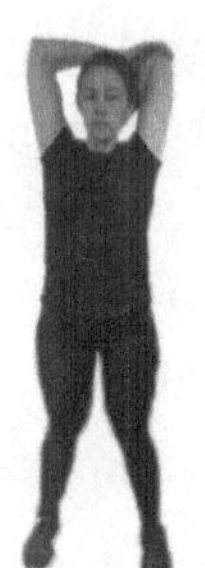

- Standing straight with your feet shoulder width apart.
- Lift your arm straight up and bend behind it backwards at the elbow.
- use opposite hand to pull the elbow snuggly towards your ear.
- Hold for 20-30 seconds and repeat with opposite side.

## <u>Abdominals</u>

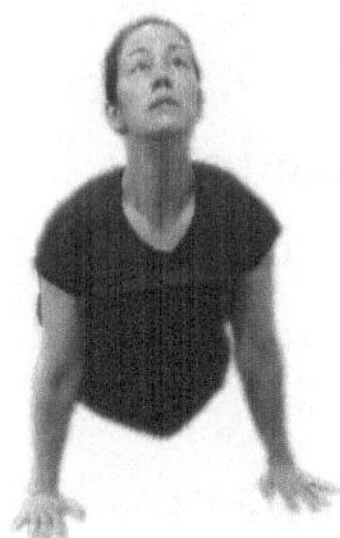

- Start by lying face down
- Put your palms flat on the floor at chest level and push your upper body off the floor
- Hold for 20-30 seconds

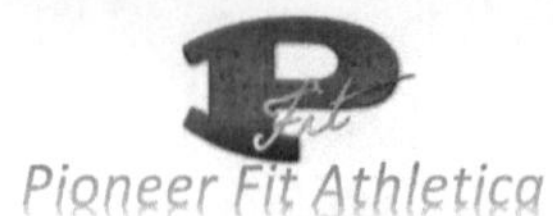


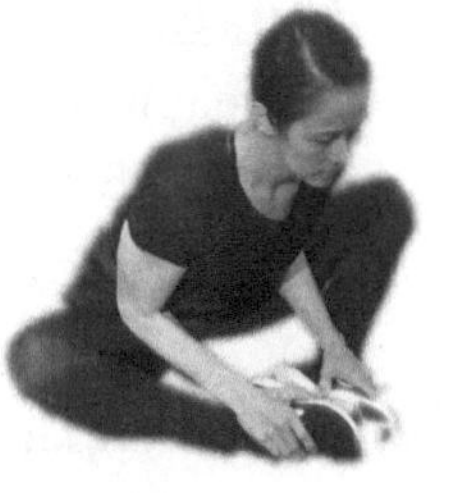

## Adductors

- Sit on floor and bend your knees, placing the balls of your feet flat against each other.
- Keeping your back straight, bend slightly forward with your hands on your ankle in as close towards you as possible.

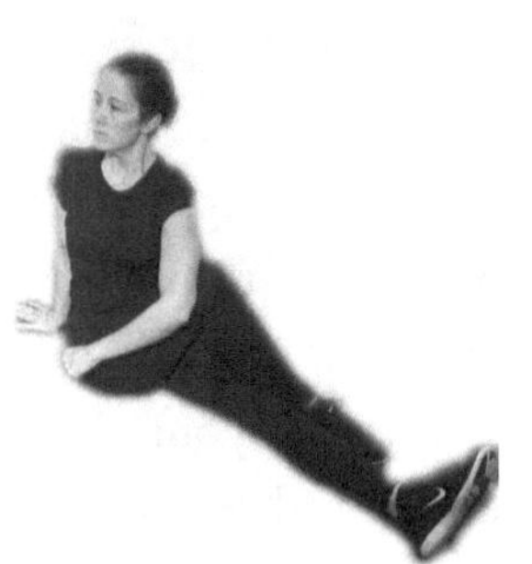

## Glutes/ Oblique

- Sit on floor with feet extended in front of you.
- Bend your right knee and place your right foot on the left of your left knee.
- Twist your body to the right and place your left had besides your right glute
- Hold for 20-30 seconds.

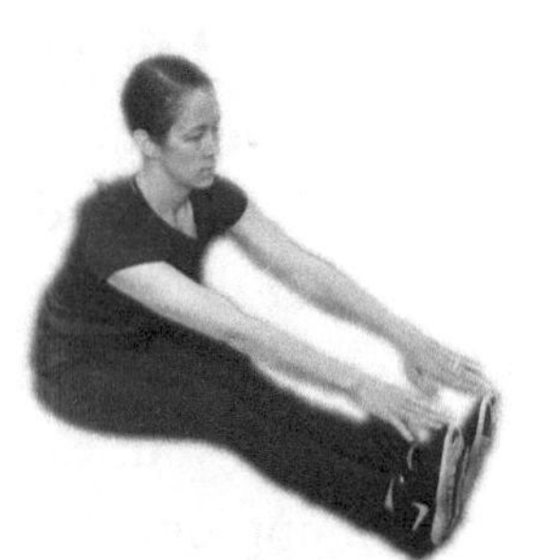

## Hamstring

- Sit with legs straight out in front
- Keeping back as straight as you can
- Lean forward from the hips and extend arms towards toes
- Hold for 20-30 seconds

## Modified Pigeon

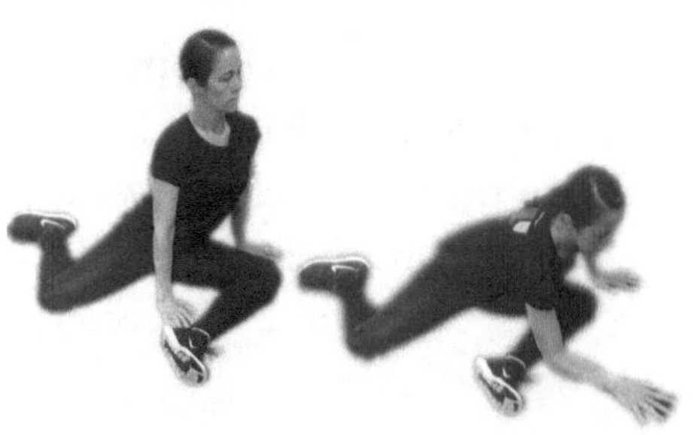

- sit on floor with one leg bent at 90* in front and the other 90* behind you.
- Lean forward from the hips keeping your back as straight as possible.

- Place opposite elbow and forearm in front of the bent leg
  - Hold for 20-30 seconds and repeat on other leg.

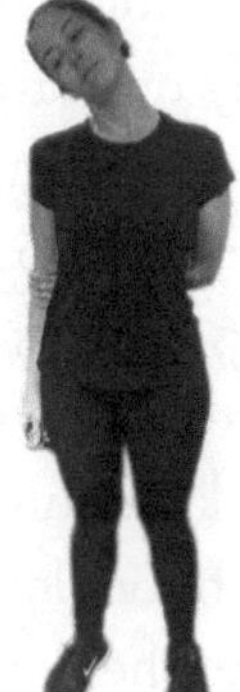

## Neck / Shoulder

- Standing straight up place one arm behind your back.
- Lean your head in the direction that the arm is going
  - Hold for 20-30 seconds and repeat on other side.

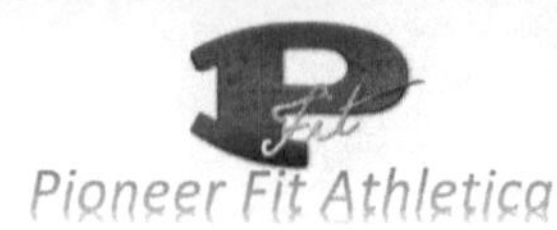
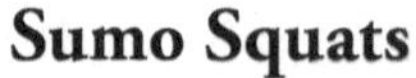
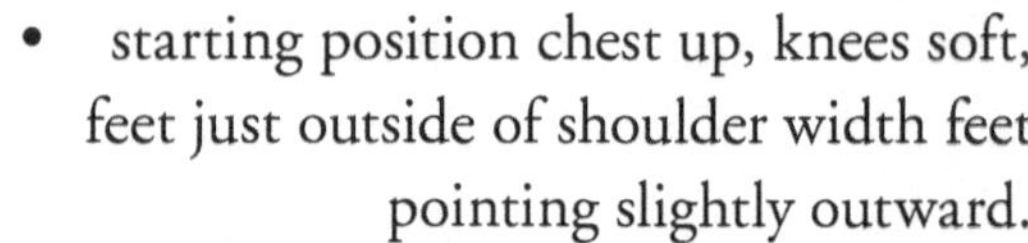



## Sumo Squats

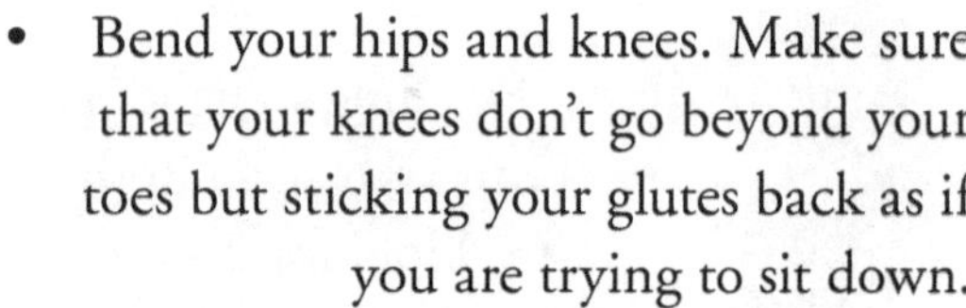

- starting position chest up, knees soft, feet just outside of shoulder width feet pointing slightly outward.
- Bend your hips and knees. Make sure that your knees don't go beyond your toes but sticking your glutes back as if you are trying to sit down.
- Continue bending your knees until your upper legs are parallel with the floor, bringing your glutes closer to the floor.
- Keep your back straight. Slowly press back up through your heels to your stating position and repeat.

## High knees

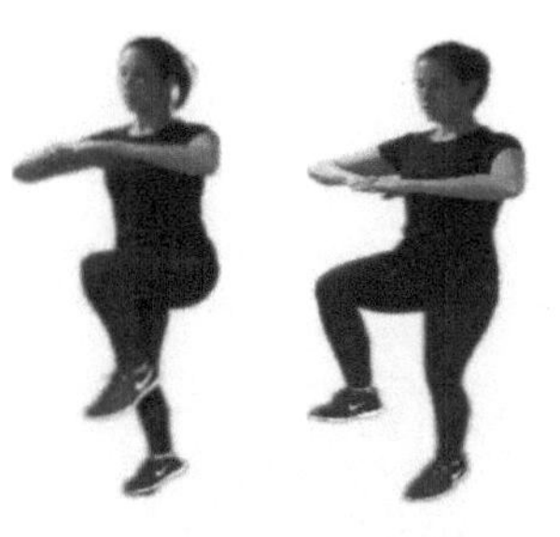

- starting position: start by standing with your feet shoulder width apart and hands by your side.
- Lift your right knee to your chest and in close succession bring your left knee to hit your palms.
- Repeat as per time/reps in workout.
- The high knee exercise is an over exaggerated jog in place with more emphasis on pulling the knees higher than your hips.

## Butt Kicks

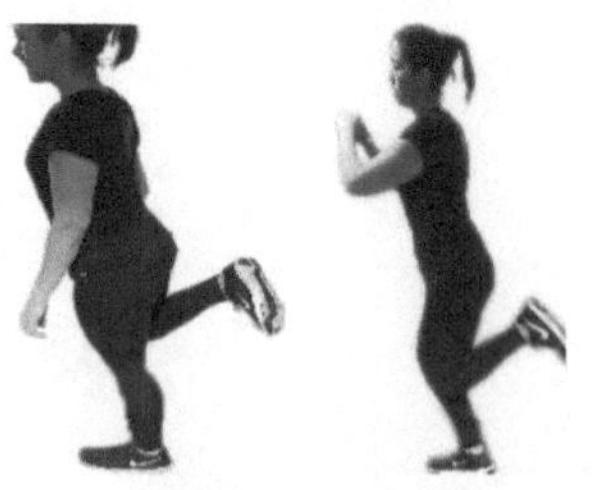

- Start off by standing straight with your feet shoulder width apart

- Kick your right foot back, bringing the heel all the way back to the butt and, in quick succession, repeat with your left leg.
- Let your arms swing or hold in front of your body for more core work.

## Leg Scissors

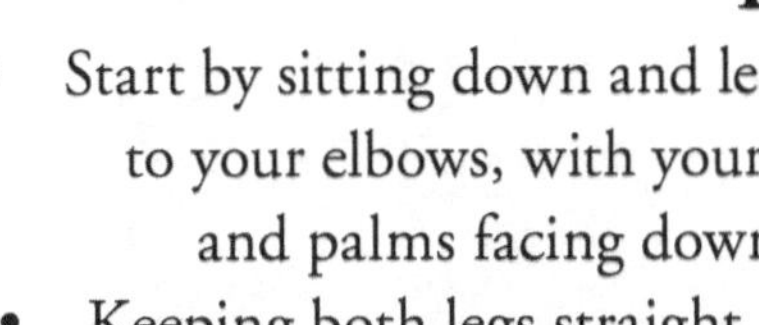

- Start by sitting down and leaning back on to your elbows, with your legs extended and palms facing down by your side.
- Keeping both legs straight, lift your right leg slightly while lifting your left leg higher than your right
- Switch positions by lifting your left leg higher that your right leg and lowering your right leg simultaneously, creating a flutter movement.
- Repeat.

## Abdominal bicycles

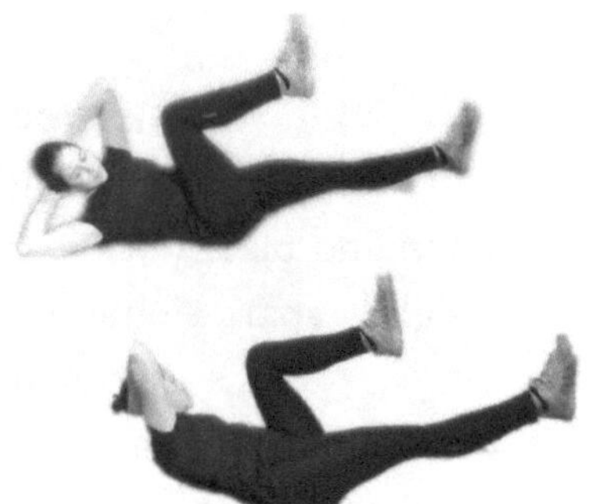

- Start by lying back on the floor or mat with your elbows bent and fingers behind your ears. Lift your shoulders off the mat.
- Bend your left knee, bringing it towards your chest while extending the right, letting it remain slightly off the ground.
- Immediately after, bring your right knee in towards the chest while extending the left to create the bike pedaling motion.

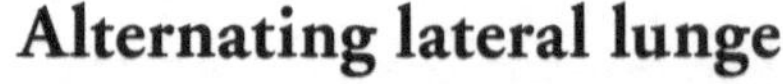

- Once you have established the movement, twist your upper body, bringing your right elbow to the left knee and vice versa.

## Alternating lateral lunge

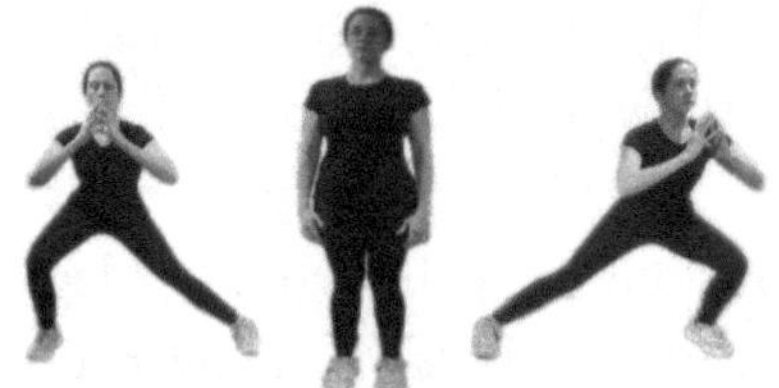

- Start off by standing with your feet shoulder width apart.
- Lift your right foot to take a large step to the right and bend your right knee about 90 degrees, lowering your body and placing your weight on your right foot.
- At the same time, prevent you knees from going beyond your toes by lowering your glutes.
- Return to your starting position by pushing straight back up through your right heel and stepping back with your right foot.
- Repeat, alternating between both legs.

## Burpee

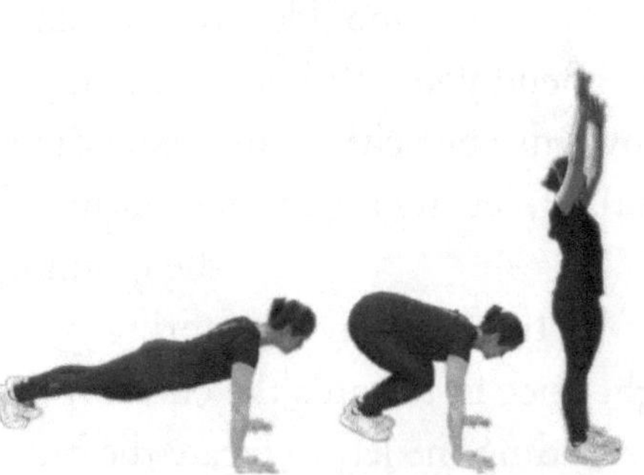

- Start in a standing position and place both feet slightly apart. Point feet outward
- Bend forward at both the hops and knees into a squatting position and place your palms flat on the floor.

- Shift your bodyweight onto your arms and kick your feet out backwards, forming a pushup position.
- Jump back into your frog jump position.
- Lift your palms and jump straight upwards or just stand, reaching your hands above your head.
- Land gently on the balls of your feet.
- Repeat.

## Jack Knives

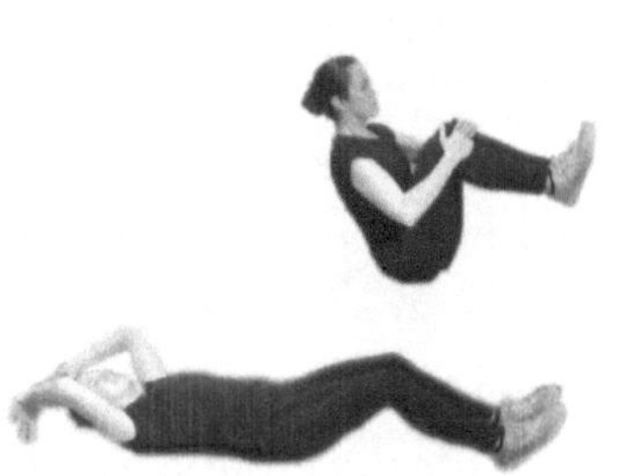

- Start by lying flat on your back with your arms extended straight behind your head and legs extended.
- Keeping your hands and legs straight, lift your upper and lower body to bring your hands towards your ankles with knees bent.
- Return to your starting position and repeat

## Mountain Climbers

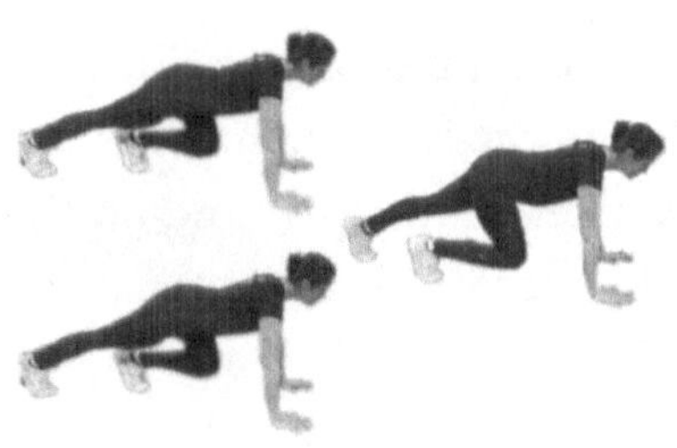

- Start in a push up position with your palms flat on the floor, shoulder width apart and your feet together.
- Bring your right knee towards your chest.
- Return your right foot to the starting position. Bring in your left knee towards your chest before returning it to the starting position.
- Repeat and gradually increase in speed.

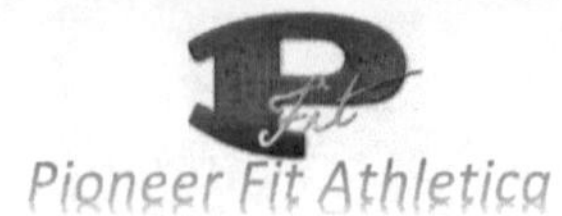


## Plank Jacks

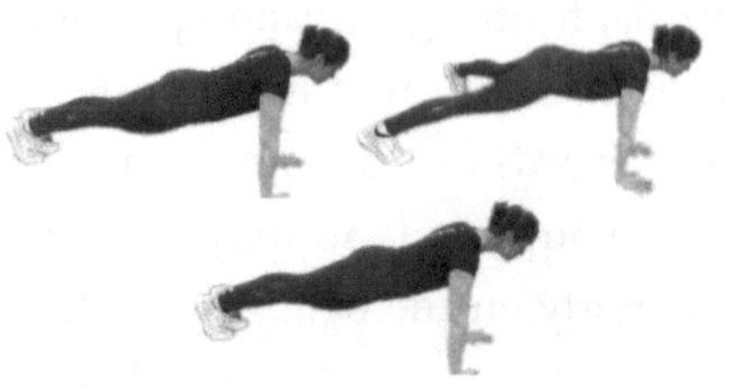

- Start off in a push up position with your feet together and palms down shoulder width apart.
- Jump your feet apart to the sides, landing on your toes and then bring it back together before repeating.

## Plank Leg Lifts

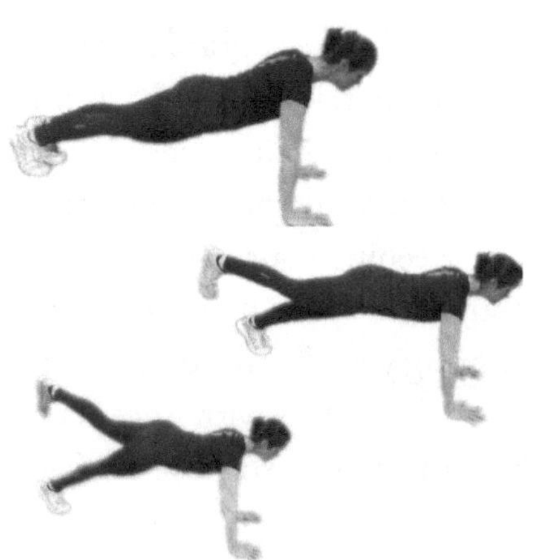

- Start in a push up position on the balls of your feet and on your elbows, instead of palms, shoulder width apart. Keep your back straight.
- Keeping our leg straight, lift your right leg off the ground as far as possible and hold.
- Return to our starting position and repeat with your left leg.

## Push ups

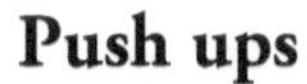

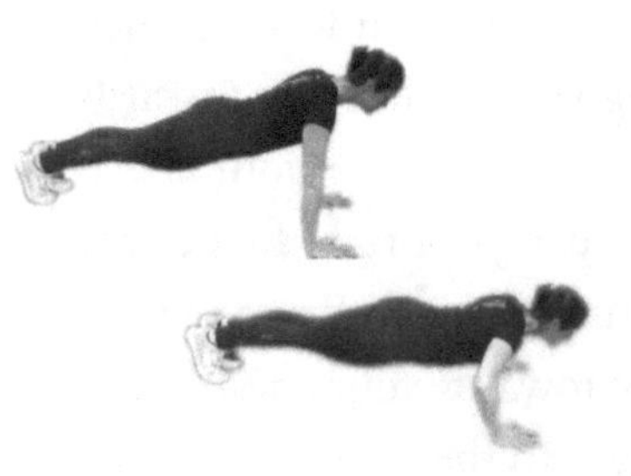

- Start in a push up position with your palms flat on the floor slightly further than shoulder width apart and on the balls of your feet, feet slightly apart.
- Keeping your back straight and in line with your glutes, bend your elbows and lower your upper body to the floor.
- Push your arms straight and return to your starting position.
- Repeat.

## Bungee

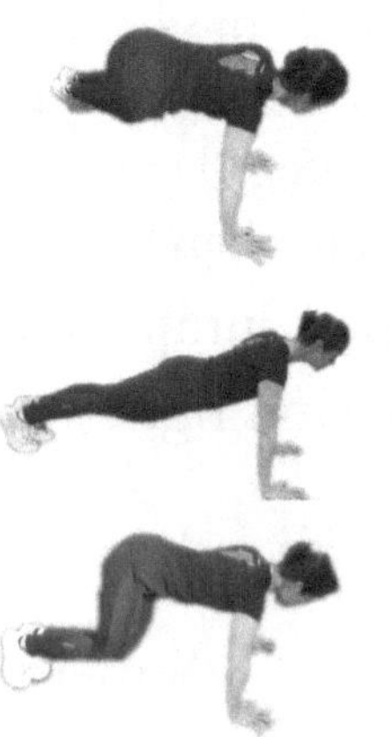

- Start in a push up position with your palms shoulder width apart and your feet together.
- Shift your bodyweight onto your arms. Keeping your palms on the floor and feet together, jump your feet to the right by bending your knees and hips.
- Repeat by jumping between left and right sides of your body.
- Repeat alternating between left and right sides of your body.

## Lateral Shuffles

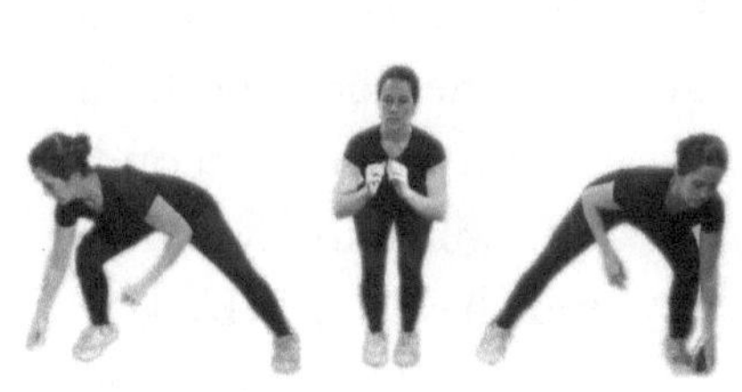

- Start off standing straight with your feet shoulder width apart and arms by your side. Bend your legs at the knees while driving your hips back slightly.
- Take a step to the right with your right foot and quickly bring your left foot to your right. As your left foot takes its step, quickly take another step to the right with your right foot. Close the distance between your feet by bringing your left foot to your right again.
- Repeat for 4 steps in the opposite direction.

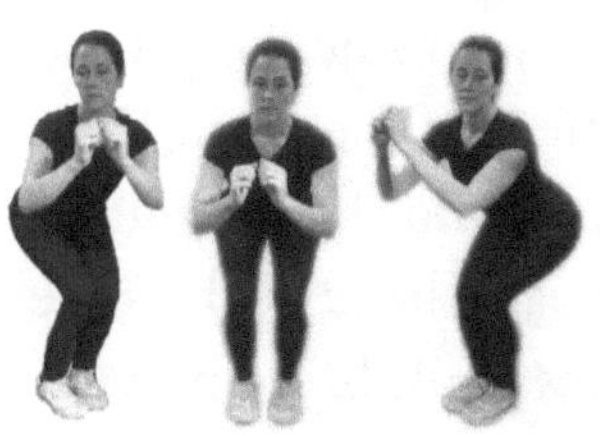

## Ski bumps

- Start in a standing position with your feet together. Bend your hips and lean

forward slightly, bed your knees. Swing both of your arms backwards.
- As you swing your arms forward, jump towards the right and land with your feet sill together and body still bent at the hips and knees.
- Swing your arms backwards and repeat jump towards the left. Alternate from left and right jumps.

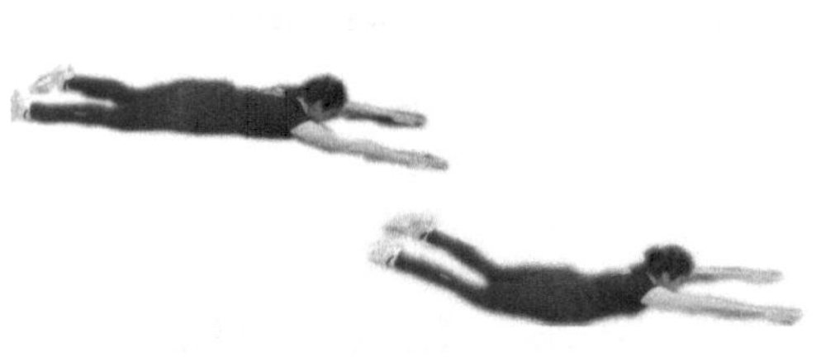

## Superman

- Start off by lying face down on the floor or mat with your arms fully extended in front of you with your legs extended as well.
- Lift your legs, chest and arms off the floor and hold for about 1 second.
- Lower your legs, arms and chest slowly back to starting position.
- Repeat.

## V ups

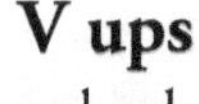
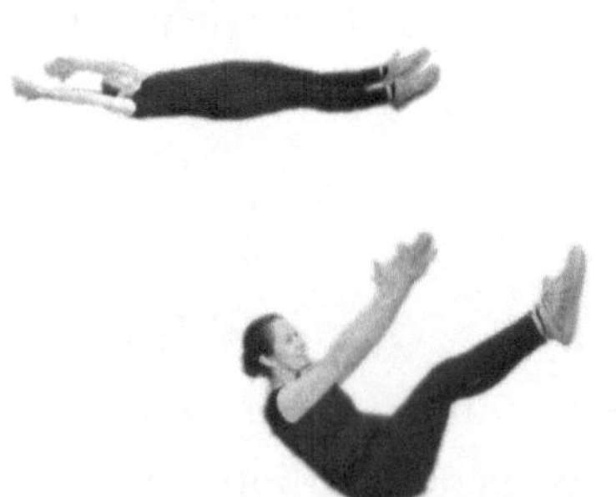

- Starting by lying on your back with your feet extended and slightly lifted off the floor. Keep your arms extended by your side. Your head should be lifted off the floor. Keep your back straight.
- Lift your feet and bend at the knee about 90 degrees while bringing your

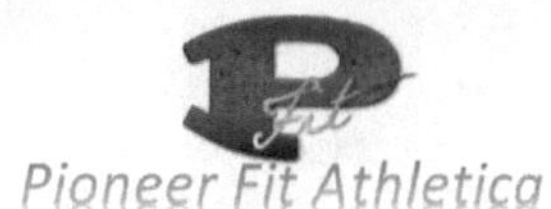


upper body as close as possible towards your legs. Keep your back straight the entire time.

- Repeat for time or reps as per workout.

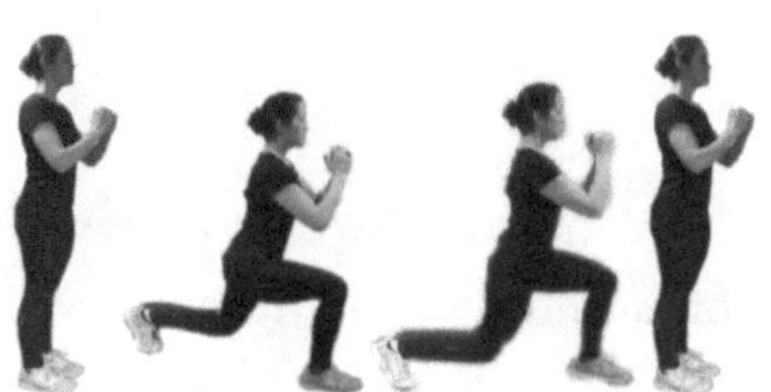

## Walking lunges

- Start off standing straight with your feet shoulder width apart and hands on your hips.
- Take a big step forward with your left foot. As you plant your left foot on the floor, bend both knees at approximately 90 degrees.
- As you extend both knees, transfer your weight completely to your left foot and take a large step forward with your right foot.
- As you plant your right foot, bend both knees at approximately 90 degrees.
- Extend both knees and transfer your weight completely onto your foot.
- And repeat.

## Triceps Dips

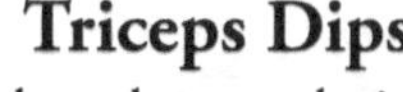

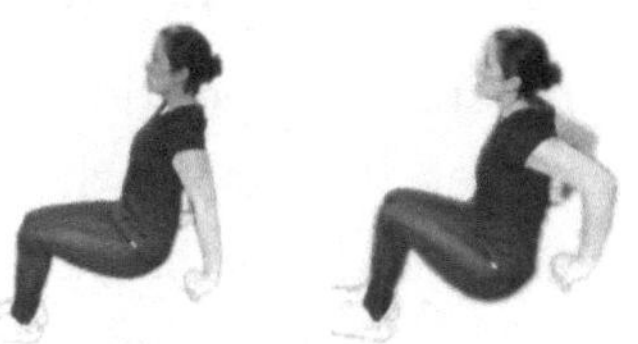

- Grip the edge of a bench or a chair with both hands at either side of you.
- Slide your body off the seat with your knees bent 90 degrees to the floor. Your

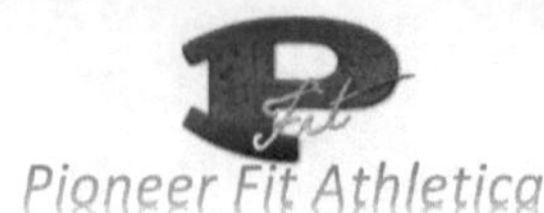



arms should be straight. This is the starting position.

- Slowly bend your elbows to lower your body towards the floor until your elbows are at about a 90degree angle. Be sure to keep your back straight and close to the bench.
- Push up through your palm of your hand. Raise your body, straightening your elbows and return to your starting position

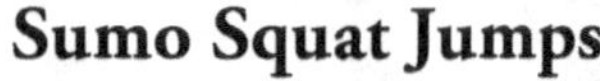

## Sumo Squat Jumps

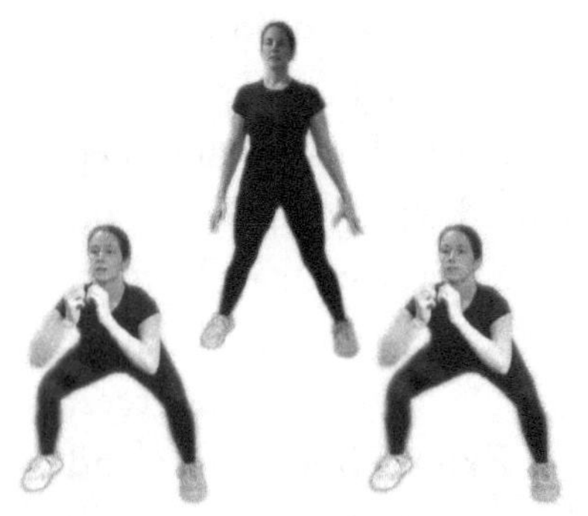

- Start off standing straight with feet shoulder width apart and hands on your hips. Point feet slightly outward.
- Bend your hips and knees. Make sure that your knees don't go beyond your toes but sticking your glues back as if you are trying to sit down.
- Continue bending your knees until your thighs are parallel with the floor, brining your glutes closer to the floor. Keep your back straight.
- Jump up, pushing your body upwards and extending your legs before landing back into squat position. Land gently on the balls of your feet.

## Split jump

- Start In a standing position
- Take a huge step forward with your right leg and bend your knee 90 degrees

- Shift your body weight onto your right leg.
- Jump into another lunge position moving your left leg in front of your right.
- Repeat

## Squat touch jump turns

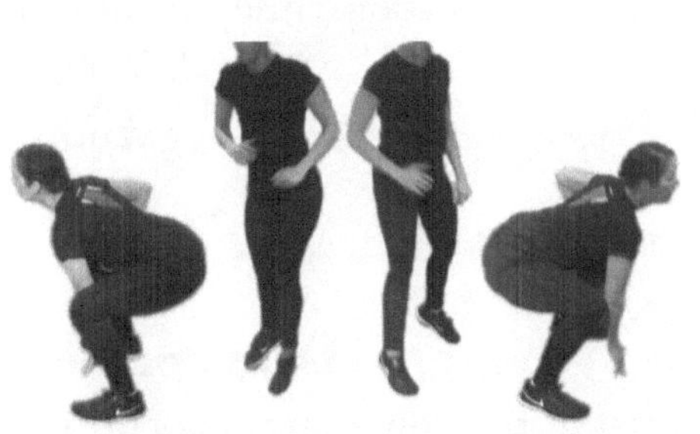

- Start in standing position with feet shoulder width apart.
- Squat down touch the ground then jump turning your body 180 degrees
- Bend knees and land in a squatting position touch the floor and repeat

## Donkey kicks

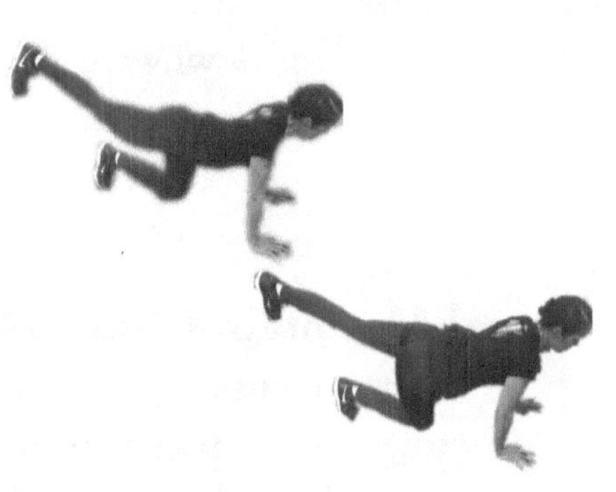

- Start off with your palms and knees on the floor
- Extend your right leg straight out behind you squeezing the glute
- Keep leg parallel to the ground pull knee back under hips and repeat.
- Repeat movement on left leg

## Switch Kicks

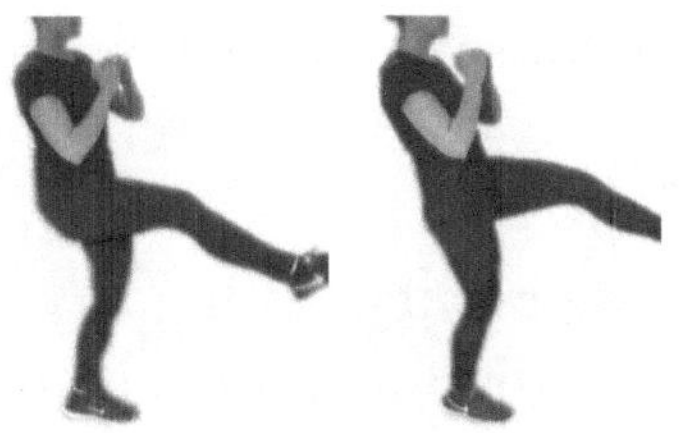

- Start in standing position
- Pick up your left leg and kick it out in front of your body

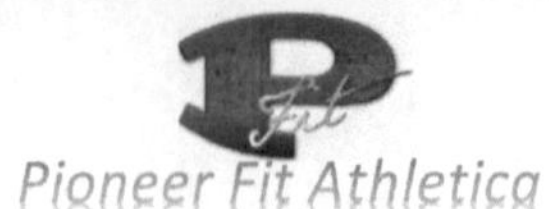
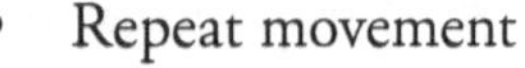


- While lowering the leg hop on to your left leg while raising your right
  - Repeat movement

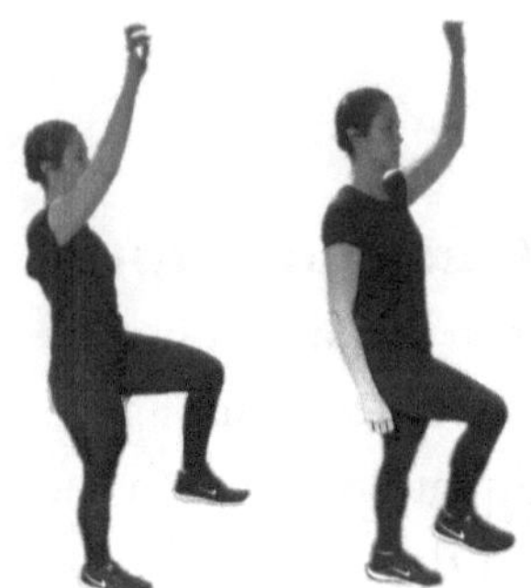

## Ladder Climbers
- Start in a standing position
- raise right hand and left knee
- Hop on to the left foot while raising the left hand
- Repeat the hoping motion

## Dive bombers

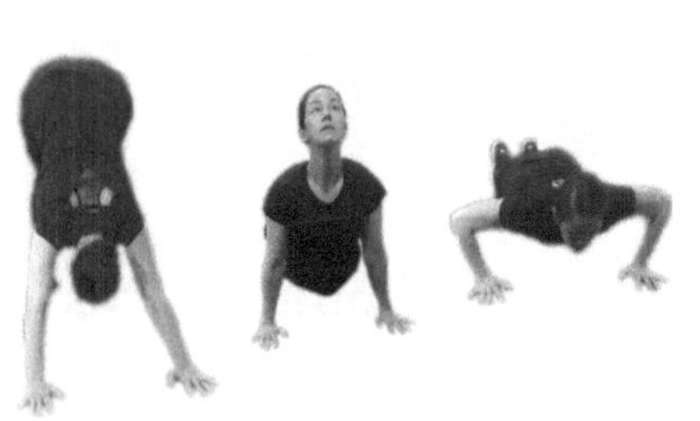

- start in the downward dog position
- Move yourself down into a pushup position
- Press your chest up and through the arms lifting the head and chin high
- Return to the downward dog position and repeat

## Rotational Mountain Climbers

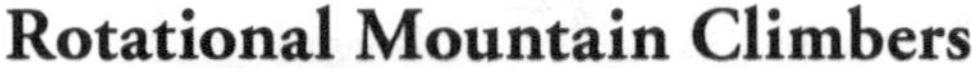
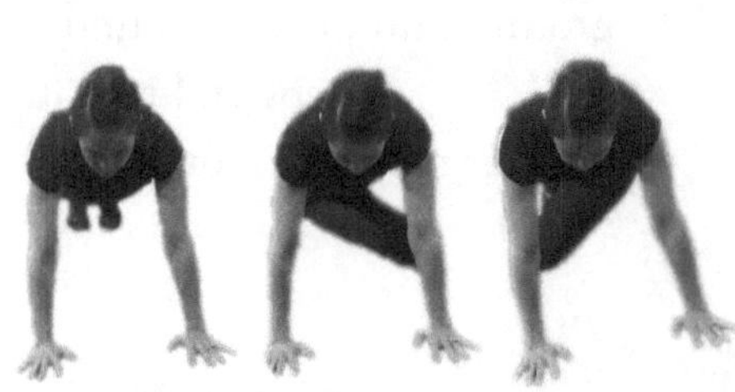

- Start in a push up position with your palms flat on the floor, shoulder width apart and your feet together.
- Bring your right knee towards your chest and across mid line.
- Return your right foot to the starting position. Bring in your left knee towards your chest and

across mid line, before returning it to the starting position.
- Repeat and gradually increase in speed

## Modified Plank Hip Rotation

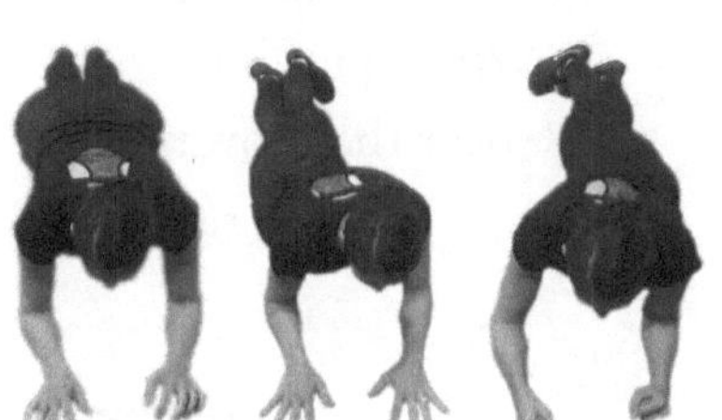

- Starting on your elbows and toes
- Rotate hips to the right allowing your hip to touch the floor
- Return to starting position, Rotate the hips towards the left allowing hip to touch floor.
- Repeat movement

## Modified Plank Alternating arm Raise

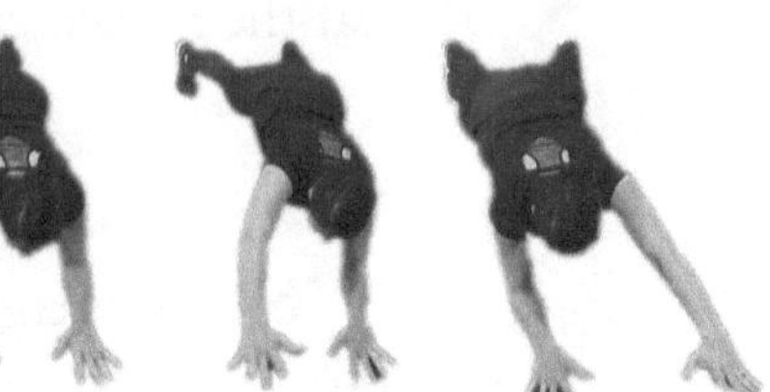

- Starting on your elbows and toes
- Shift weight to the left elbow while raising right hand.
- Lower arm and shift weight to the right elbow
- Lift the left hand and repeat movement.

## Glute Bridge

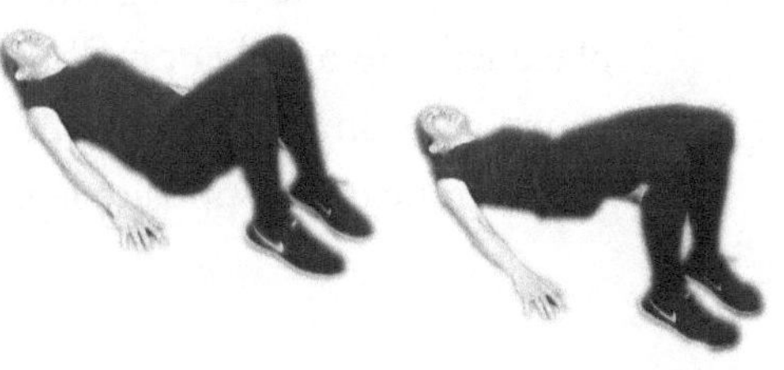

- Start off by lying on your back on the floor with your knees bent and your palms facing down, by your sides.
- Pushing with your heels, lift your hips off the floor.

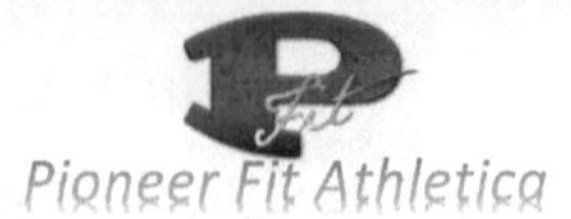
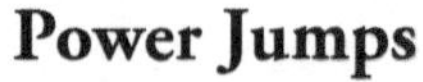


## Power Jumps

- Start in the quarter squat position
- Explode up into a jump bringing the knees up
- While the knees are rising up touch the top of knees with open hands
- Land as soft as possible in the quarter squat position.
- Repeat the movement

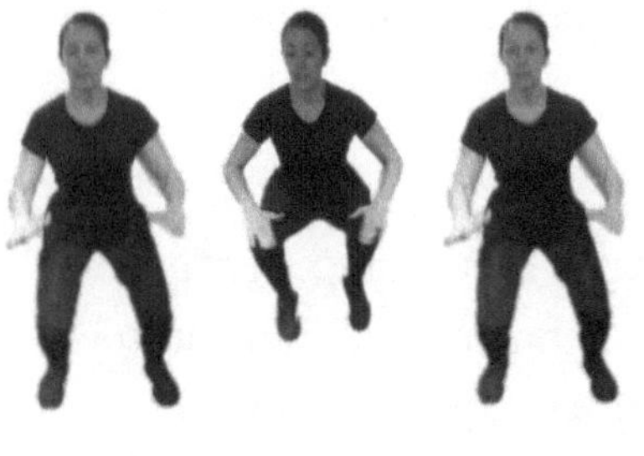

## Froggers

- Start in the full squat position
- Touch the floor with both hands
- Explode into a squat jump, pushing your body forward
- Land in a full squat and touch the floor
- Repeat the movement

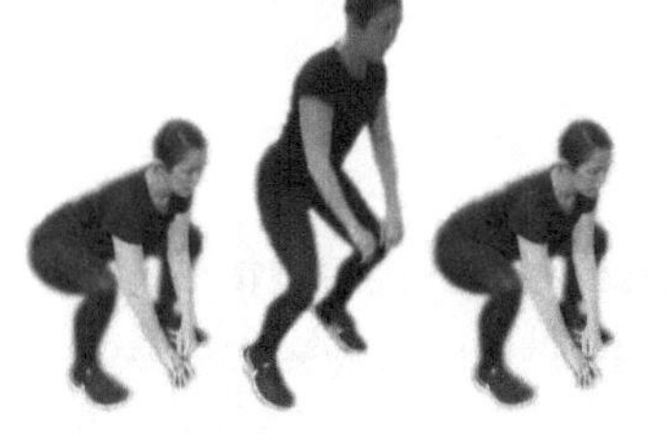

## Sit through

- Start in the pushup position feet together
- Pull your right knee to hip height
- Pull the leg across the body extend the leg then place left hip and leg on floor
- Once the hip touches the floor return to pushup position and repeat on opposite leg.

## Jumping jacks

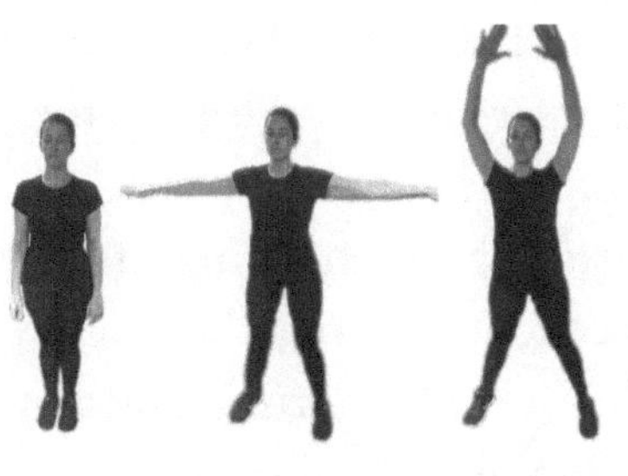

- Start in a standing position with feet together hands at sides
- Hop feet out away from each other while bringing arms away from your sides to the overhead position.
- Hop the feet back together while lowering the arms back down to the side.
- Repeat the movement

## Robot pushups

- Starting in a pushup position
- Lower your right elbow to the floor
- Followed by your left elbow
- Then place right palm on floor pushing your upper body up
- Followed up by the left palm to the floor returning you back to the starting position.
- Repeat on both sides

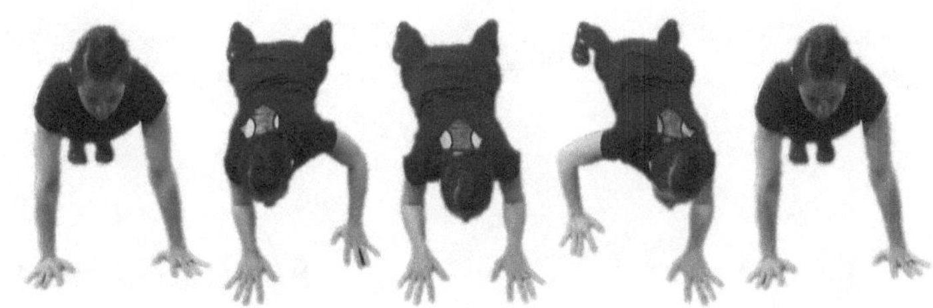

## Seated rotation

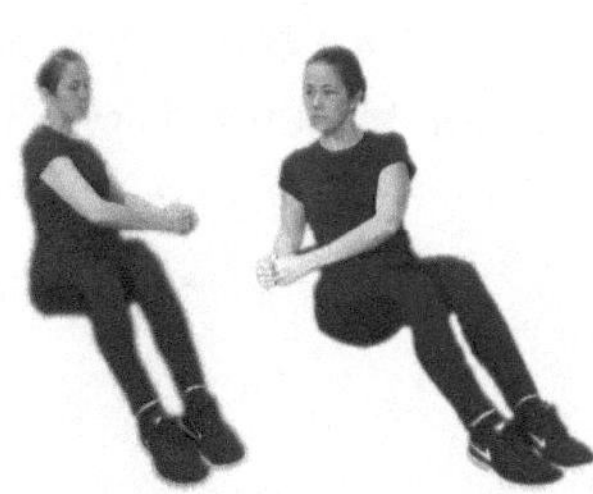

- Start in seated position with knees bent in front of you.
- clasp hands together and twist your body to reach over to your right and try to touch the ground.
- Repeat on both sides.

## Plank alternating knee

- Start in a push up position with your palms flat on the floor, shoulder width apart and your feet together.
- Bring your right knee towards your chest.
- Return your right foot to the starting position. Bring in your left knee towards your chest before returning it to the starting position.
- Repeat and pause each knee.

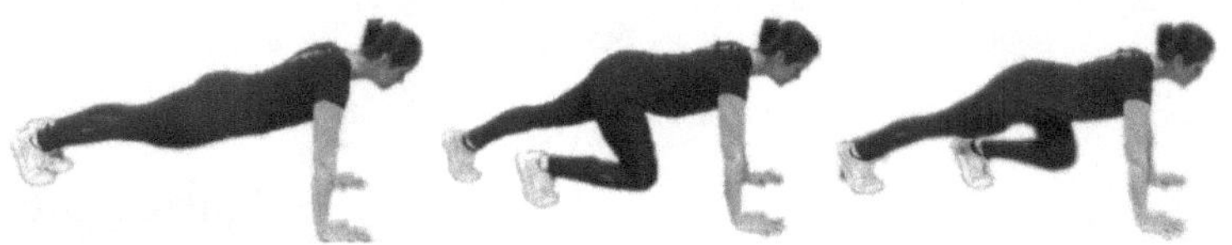

## Push up jacks

- Starting in the push up position with feet apart
- Hop feet together and bend elbows into a push up, then hop feet apart returning to the push up position.
- Repeat the pattern

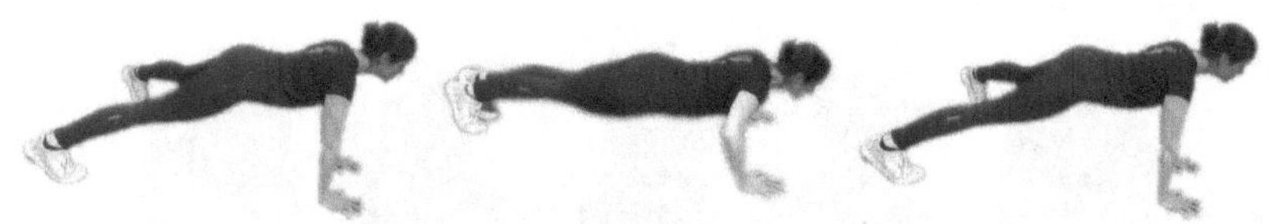

## Front and back hops

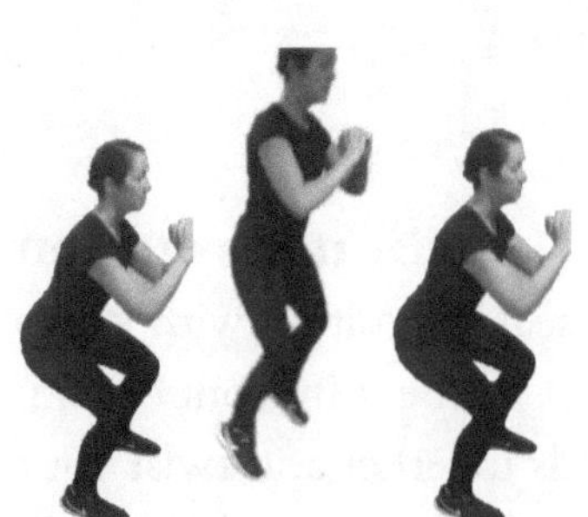

- Start in the squat position
- Hop forward about two feet, landing into squat position.
- Once landed, hop back wards two feet landing in the squat position.
- Repeat

## 123 knee

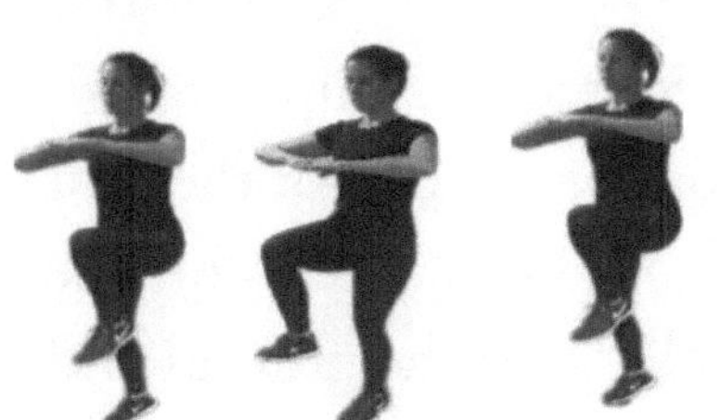

- Start in standing position.
- Perform three high knee moving lateral.
- Once the third knee is done return to the opposite side for
- three lateral knee.

## Lateral Towel jumps

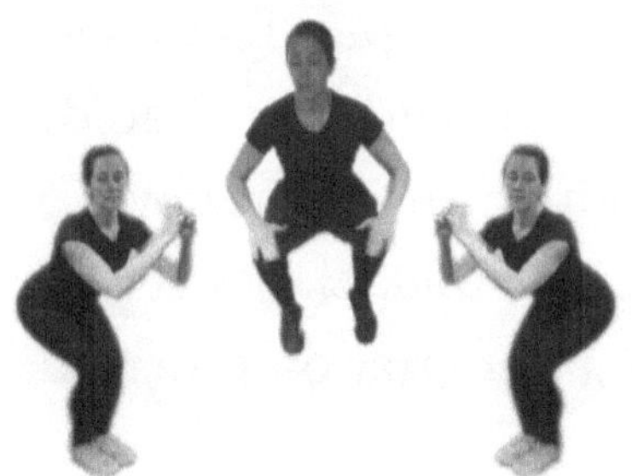

- start in bent knee position standing beside towel
- hop with both feet laterally over the towel
- landing with knees bent
- repeat

## Plank shoulder touches

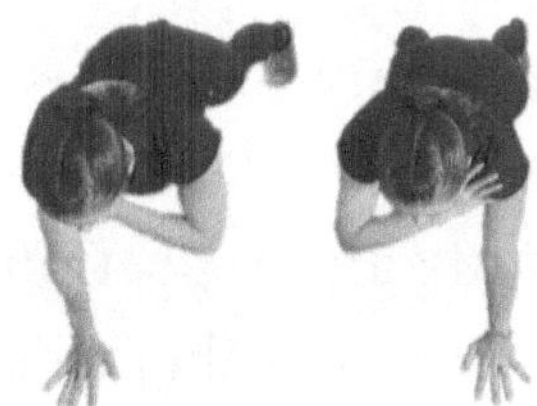

Start off in pushup position
Alternate hands touching opposite
Shoulder.

## Flutter kicks

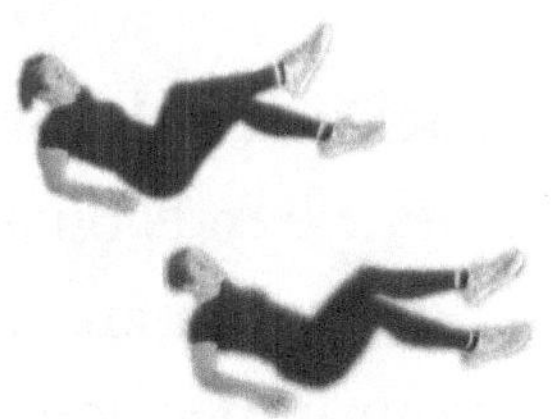

Start resting on elbows
Knees bent, alternate raising each leg
Take your time and try not to raise
legs too high.

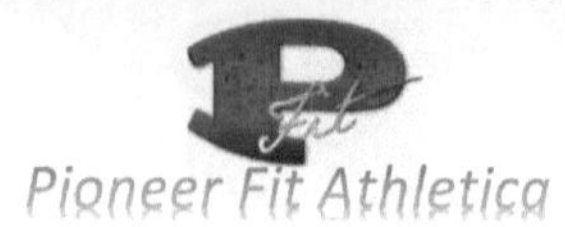


## Calf Raise

Start standing flat footed Push up through the toes or the pad of the foot raising heals off the Floor, return back to the ground and repeat.

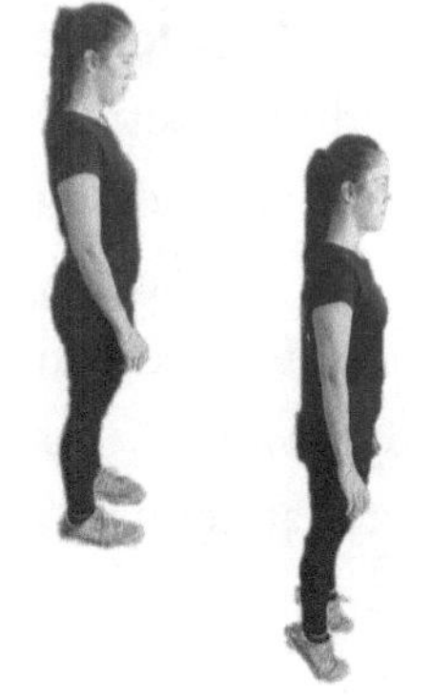

## squat front kick

Start with feet shoulder width apart squat down as you come up kick one leg out front and repeat on other side

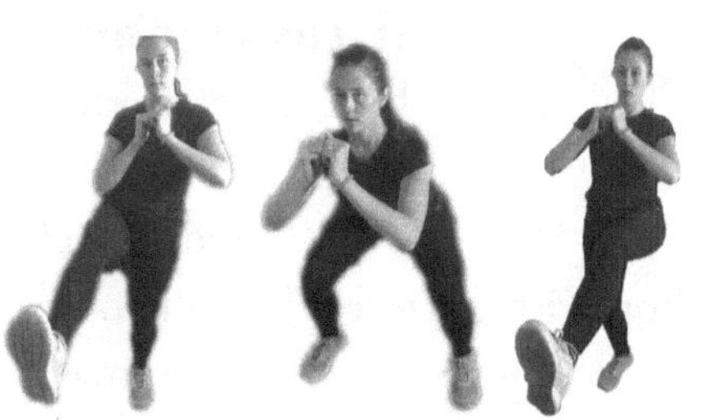

## Squat side kick

Start with feet shoulder width apart squat down as you come up kick one leg out laterally and repeat on other side

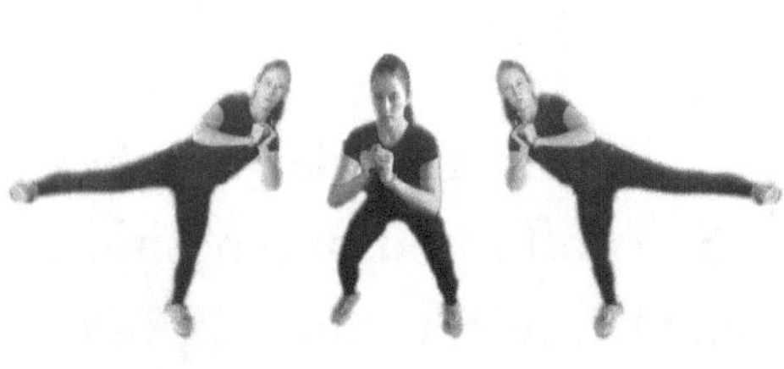

## Incline pushups

Start with your hands on a bench shoulder width apart Lower your upper body down toward hands Push upper body up to starting to position

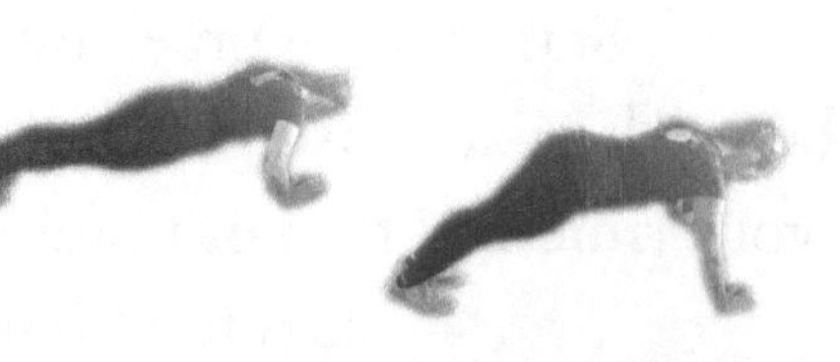

## Pulse Squat/Pioneer Squats
start with feet shoulder width apart
squat down to comfort and pause
then come up slightly
then back down
repeat.

www.ingramcontent.com/pod-product-compliance
Lightning Source LLC
Chambersburg PA
CBHW051449250726
48655CB00001B/328